SIXTH EDITION

FITNESS
FOR THE HEALTH OF IT

RUTH LINDSEY
CALIFORNIA STATE UNIVERSITY
LONG BEACH

BILLIE J. JONES
FLORIDA STATE UNIVERSITY
TALLAHASSEE

ADA VAN WHITLEY
OKLAHOMA STATE UNIVERSITY
STILLWATER

wcb
Wm. C. Brown Publishers
Dubuque, Iowa

Cover design by Laurie Entringer.

Library of Congress Catalog Card Number: 88–70350

ISBN 0–697–07282–7

Printed in the United States of America by Wm. C. Brown Publishers 2460 Kerper Boulevard, Dubuque, IA 52001

10 9 8 7 6

Contents

List of Tables

Preface

Fitness for the Health of It is a revision of the text which was originally named *Body Mechanics* and was called *Fitness: Health, Figure/Physique, Posture* in the fifth edition. The change in title for the sixth edition reflects the focus on being totally fit because it is the healthy thing to do. It continues to be designed for young adult men and women, but the materials and information are suitable for anyone high school age and older.

The basic topics are the same as in earlier editions; however, the information has been expanded and updated. Chapters have been reordered and a new one, Fitness Programs, included. Questions are posed at the beginning of each chapter. There are more tables, illustrations, and tests, and a glossary has been added.

The text remains a workbook that is designed primarily for an exercise course. The emphasis is on "do-it-yourself" with tests and measurements for evaluating current status, suggestions for setting personal goals, and the means for accomplishing these goals.

An *Instructor's Manual* which accompanies this text includes a course outline and additional exercises and resources. It contains suggested materials for testing and teaching—such as stunts, games, demonstrations, equipment needed, and a list of resources—to add variety to class presentations.

We would like to express our gratitude to our colleagues who have used prior editions of this text for providing comments and suggestions, many of which have been incorporated into this sixth edition. We would also like to thank the reviewers who worked with us on this edition: Buck Jones, University of Tennessee, Knoxville; Carol L. Doenges, Olivet Nazarene University; Paulette Walker Johnson, Virginia State University; and Linda Velvin Narisi, University of Central Arkansas.

D. R. L.
B. J. J.
A. V. W.

Introduction

If you had a new luxury car, you would want to keep that fine machine in excellent condition by performing regular preventive maintenance on it. You would use only the best fuel in it and you would drive it regularly to prevent the parts from becoming corroded and to keep them running smoothly. You would not dream of parking it in the garage and just letting it rust, nor would you put french perfume in the gas tank or run it without air in the tires or oil in the crank case!

No, most of us would not think of abusing or misusing an expensive car, but many of us do it to our bodies. The human body is often referred to as the "human machine." With its 206 bones and 639 muscles and miles of nerves (electrical lines) and blood vessels (fuel lines) and other tissues, it probably has more moving parts and is more complicated than most man-made machines, yet it is governed by the same mechanical principles as other machines. It too must have proper care and use and regular preventive maintenance to function efficiently. Keeping our bodies in good running condition however is far more important than preserving an automobile. *We can't trade it on a new model!!*

This book is a "preventive maintenance user's manual" for the human machine. It is a text-workbook on how to become physically fit and stay that way and how to use the body in activities of daily living to avoid strain. Chapter 1 provides tests and measurements to help you assess your present status on strength, neuromuscular endurance, flexibility, cardiovascular endurance, body composition, weight, and figure/physique proportions. The second chapter introduces the concept of physical fitness and distinguishes between health-related and skill-related fitness; it discusses the importance of exercise in terms of its immediate effects as well as its long term benefits.

Chapter 3, probably the "heart" of the text, provides the theoretical foundations for developing an exercise program and gives general suggestions to help you get a maximum of benefit and enjoyment from exercise. The role of exercise for the purpose of improving one's appearance is discussed in addition to conditioning for fitness. Because many books and magazines and unqualified leaders advise you to perform exercises that are potentially harmful, some questionable exercises are described in this chapter along with advice to avoid them or modify them to prevent injury. The fourth chapter provides a practical "how-to-do-it" approach with suggestions for exercise. It includes aerobic exercise, progressive resistance exercise, calisthenics, and weight training for fitness improvement; also, selected exercises for specific body parts are described for those who wish to concentrate on figure/physique problems.

A variety of fitness programs are examined in chapter 5, including walking, rope jumping, swimming, cycling, Canadian XBX, aerobic exercise, and selected sports. Chapter 6 discusses body composition and distinguishes between weight and fatness. Several screening techniques which have been recommended by the National Institutes of Health are explained and interpreted, including abdominal/hip girth ratio, body mass index, skinfolds, and relative weight. The importance of proper body composition and the dangers of bulemia and anorexia are discussed. Good nutrition is described and the role of diet and exercise in weight/fat control is explained. Tables are provided to show the number of calories used in selected exercise and the number of calories in food (including fast foods). Suggestions for both gaining and losing weight are given.

There are quacks in every profession and the fitness and exercise business is no exception, as chapter 7 makes clear. Our laws are woefully inadequate to protect us from rip-offs and incompetency—so our only protection is being educated consumers. Toward that end, this chapter exposes a few examples of nutritional fads, reducing drugs, gadgets, and gimmicks, and some fallacies and misconceptions about weight/fat control and exercise.

Chapter 8 defines good and bad posture and discusses the importance of the proper alignment of body parts. Suggestions are provided for how to achieve good posture, how to stand in good alignment and how to use efficient body mechanics during activities of daily living, including ascending and descending stairs, and sitting and rising. Chapter 9 explains how to protect the spine. It has been estimated that 93,000,000 workdays per year are lost because of backaches, and sooner or later, most of us will end up in a doctor's office with an aching back. Because of the prevalence of this disability, we discuss its causes and give some guidelines for preventing back and neck aches. Since spine problems are often caused by using poor body mechanics, proper methods of lifting, carrying, pushing, and pulling are described. Specific exercises are included for preventing or alleviating back problems.

In addition to backaches most of us will also suffer from aching feet at sometime in our lives. Since walking, jogging, and aerobic exercise have become so popular, there is an even greater need to know how to take care of your feet. Chapter 10 describes how to choose proper shoes (including jogging and aerobic shoes). Common foot and leg problems are discussed and specific exercises for the feet and legs are described.

Chapter 11 discusses some of the causes and effects of neuromuscular hypertension and provides some suggestions for preventing chronic tension build-up. Several healthy ways of releasing tension are included and a conscious relaxation technique is described in detail, along with a few exercises designed for tension release. Finally, chapter 12 is aimed primarily at women. The focus is on the role of exercise in dysmenorrhea, pregnancy, and osteoporosis.

The Appendix contains workbook-types of tear-out charts and other supplementary material designed to accompany the chapters. The charts make it possible for the reader to record pre- and post-test scores on fitness, posture, and foot alignment. There are charts for goal setting and recording of progress; a nutrition pre-test; charts for recording daily and weekly caloric intake; and charts for graphing weight changes. Documentation of accomplishment can be rewarding.

We hope that you will read and heed the information in these chapters with success and joy. Inactivity, along with aging, will cause negative changes in your musculoskeletal and cardiorespiratory systems. This book offers a wide range of suggestions so that your machine can avoid "body rust" and you can be fit for the health of it!

Assessing Your Status

1

PRETEST

1. How do you decide if you should get a physical exam before starting an exercise program?
2. How do you warm up and cool down?
3. Why should you measure your physical fitness status before beginning an exercise program?
4. How can you measure your present fitness status?
5. What can you learn from skinfold measurements?
6. What are the three basic types of body builds?

HEALTH SCREENING

Before initiating a program of self-improvement, you need to assess your present status. For most people, participating in physical activity should not pose any problem or health hazard, but there is a small number of adults for whom physical activity might be inappropriate or those who should have medical advice concerning the type of activity most suitable for them. To prevent having to undergo unnecessary medical exams, answer the following questions from the Par-Q Test.[1]

1. Has your doctor ever said you have heart trouble?
2. Do you frequently have pain in your heart and chest?
3. Do you often feel faint or have spells of dizziness?
4. Has a doctor ever said your blood pressure was too high?
5. Has a doctor ever told you that you have a bone or joint problem such as arthritis that has been aggravated by exercise or might be made worse with exercise?
6. Is there a good physical reason not mentioned here why you should not follow an activity program even if you wanted to?
7. Are you over age 65 and not accustomed to vigorous exercise?

If you answered YES to one or more of these questions, consult with your personal physician before increasing your physical activity and/or taking a fitness test and tell the doctor which questions you answered YES. After medical evaluation, follow your physician's recommendation regarding any restrictions in your physical activity.

If you answered NO to all of the questions accurately, you have reasonable assurance of your present suitability for a graduated exercise program. If you have a temporary illness, such as a cold, you may wish to postpone physical activity.

WARM-UP AND COOL-DOWN

Before embarking on an exercise program or on tests of your physical fitness, you should stretch and warm up; at the end of vigorous exercise, you should cool down and stretch again. Most experts believe this precaution will help prevent some muscular soreness or possibly injury.

Warm up by performing some mild stretching of the major muscle groups, particularly the ones you are most apt to use in the activity. Increase the circulation of your heart muscle as well as your skeletal muscles by performing some mild cardiovascular activity such as walking and arm swinging, jogging, swimming, or cycling for two or three minutes. The cool-down may consist of the same activities you used in the warm-up, except the skeletal muscles which were used most vigorously should be stretched statically in your target zone for flexibility.

If you have been sedentary for several weeks, you may wish to practice the exercises in this chapter for three or four weeks before taking these maximal effort tests to avoid undue muscular soreness.

FITNESS, PHYSIQUE, AND FIGURE ANALYSIS

This chapter describes a battery of tests which measures samples of the health-related aspects of your physical fitness: muscular endurance, cardiovascular endurance, strength, flexibility, and body composition. In addition, guidelines are provided for measuring your "shape" (figure/physique). On the basis of the results of these tests and measurements, you should set goals for yourself and design a program of exercises and activities to meet your needs. Subsequent chapters will provide guidance for this purpose.

After taking the tests, record your scores and rankings on Charts I, II, and III in the Appendix. You may wish to repeat the tests periodically to determine whether your program is effective. Chart IV (Appendix) should tell you if you are improving, so that you can revise your program if necessary. Those who are enrolled in a formal class may be asked to make a final assessment at the end of the course and record the results on Charts I, II, and III for comparison with their initial scores.

It is important that you exert maximum effort on each of the performance tests and that you follow the directions for tests and measures precisely. This will enable you to obtain a more accurate picture of your status and to compare your scores with the norms of your age group.

TESTS FOR PHYSICAL FITNESS

Test IA   Pull-ups (Arm Strength and Endurance). Hang from a bar with palms facing the body. Pull up until the chin is over the bar and then lower the body until the arms are completely extended again. Continue until you can do no more. Do not kick or twist or stay in one position for more than two seconds. Excessive swaying should be prevented by a partner. The score is the total number of pull-ups completed without stopping (up and down = 1 count).

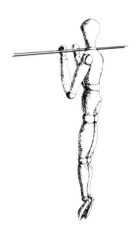

FIGURE 1.1 Pull-up and bent-arm hang

Test IB   Bent-Arm Hang (For the Person Who Can Not Execute a Pull-up Successfully). Stand on a chair and grasp the bar with palms facing the body. Have someone remove the chair while you hang with your chin over the bar (see illustration) as long as possible, up to 25 seconds. The score is the number of seconds you were able to hang.

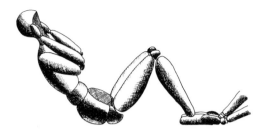

FIGURE 1.2 Crunch (curl-up)

Test II   Crunches (Curl-Up) (For Upper Abdominal Strength and Endurance). Assume a hook-lying position with your hands placed on your cheeks. Flex the head, neck, and upper trunk, rolling up *only until the lower angle of your scapulae leave the floor.* Roll down until your head touches the mat. Repeat as many times as possible in 60 seconds. (Up and down = 1 count).

Test IIIA   Push-Ups (Arm and Shoulder Strength and Endurance). Face the floor and support your body on your toes and hands while keeping the arms and the body straight and stiff. Lower the body by flexing the elbows until your chest touches the floor, then push up to the starting position. Do not allow the body to "pike" or "sag" at the hips. Count the number of correct push-ups done continuously (without rest). (Down and up = 1 count.) You may stop when you can no longer execute a correct push-up.

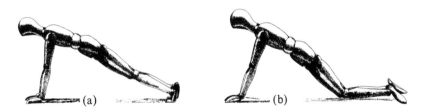

FIGURE 1.3 (a) Push-up. Note: Norms given for this test are for men. (b) Modified push-up. Note: Norms given for this test are for women.

Test IIIB   Modified Push-ups (Arm and Shoulder Strength and Endurance). Assume a modified push-up position with the hands on the floor under the shoulders, arms straight, and knees bent. Keep the body straight from head to knees, while lowering the body until the chest touches the floor. Return to the starting position. Do not allow the hips to bend (pike) or the back to sag (arch). The score is the number of correct push-ups done continuously (without rest). (Down and up = 1 count.)

Test IV Sit and Reach (Flexibility of the Lower Back and Hamstrings). Sit on the floor with the legs together and extended, and the soles of the feet against a bench, turned on its side, to which a ruler has been attached. Keep your knees straight and reach as far as you can comfortably reach, then gently stretch forward over the ruler three times. Hold the position on the third reach for three seconds minimum. Do *not* touch the ruler during the hold. The score is read in inches from the fingertips to the toes (edge of the bench). For example, if you reach to your toes, your score is 0; if you reach six inches past your toes, your score is +6″; if you lack two inches reaching your toes, your score is −2″.

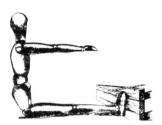

FIGURE 1.4 Sit and reach

Test V 1.5 Mile Run/Walk (Cardiovascular Endurance). On a measured track, cover the distance of a mile and a half in as short a time as possible. Try to pace yourself so you can jog the entire distance. It is permissable to walk if necessary. On a quarter-mile (one-fourth mile) track, you would run/walk six laps while being timed with a stop watch. Your score is the length of time, to the nearest second, in which you covered the distance.

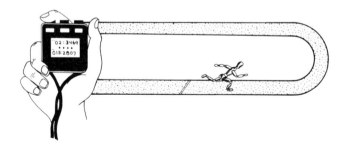

FIGURE 1.5 Run/walk 1.5 miles

MUSCULAR ENDURANCE TESTS USING WEIGHTS

If you have access to free weights or weight machines, you may wish to take these additional tests of muscular endurance. If you are in a class, these should be done under the supervision of your instructor. If you are not in a class, you should work under the guidance of a person knowledgeable about weight lifting techniques and safety.

Test VI   Biceps Curl (two-arm) (For elbow flexors, e.g., biceps). Select a resistance equivalent to one-third of your body weight. Stand with feet shoulder width apart; hold a barbell in front of the body against the thighs; place hands shoulder width apart with palms facing up (away from the body). Stabilize the trunk by contracting the abdominals and the gluteals. Flex the elbows and "curl" the forearms until they contact the upper arm, then slowly lower the weight to its starting position. Repeat continuously (no rest). Each lift = 1 count). Note: This test uses some of the same muscles as Tests 1A and 1B and should not be performed on the same day.

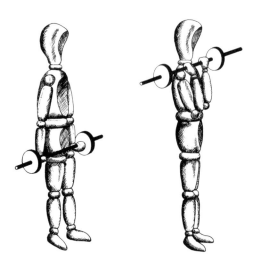

FIGURE 1.6 Biceps curl

Test VII   Bench Press (For shoulder flexors and elbow extensors e.g., pectoralis major and triceps). Select a resistance that is two-thirds of your body weight. Lie supine on the bench with the hips and knees bent and feet on the bench or on a wall. The handles should be in line with the chest. Grasp the handles with palms facing away from the face. Lift the weight by extending the elbows until they are straight (do not lock elbows), then slowly return to the starting position. Repeat continuously. (Each lift = 1 count.) Note: This test uses some of the same muscles as Tests IIIA and IIIB and should not be performed on the same day.

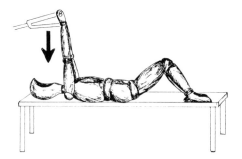

FIGURE 1.7 Bench press

Test VIII   Lat Pull-Downs (For shoulder adductors and elbow flexors, e.g., latissimus dorsi and biceps). Select a resistance two-thirds of your body weight. Assume a kneeling position under the "Lat" bar, facing the machine. Grasp the handles with the palms facing the machine. Stabilize the trunk by contracting the abdominals and gluteals. Lift the weight by pulling the bar down behind the head until it touches the base of your neck then slowly return to the starting position. Repeat continuously. (Each pull-down = 1 count.) Note: This test uses some of the same muscles as Tests IA and IB and should not be performed on the same day.

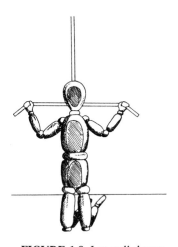

FIGURE 1.8 Lat pull-downs

Test IX Hamstring Curls (For knee flexors, e.g., hamstrings). Choose a resistance that is one third of your body weight. Lie prone on the bench with heels under the pad, cheek resting on the bench, and hands grasping sides of bench. Flex the knees, "curling" the legs until the feet are over the buttocks or the pad touches the buttocks. Slowly lower to the starting position and repeat continuously. (Each lift = 1 count.)

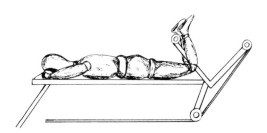

FIGURE 1.9 Hamstring curls

Test X Quadriceps Extensions (For knee extensors, e.g., quadriceps femoris). Choose a resistance that is two-thirds of your body weight. Sit on the end of the bench with ankles under the pads and hands grasping sides of the bench. Extend your knees (do not lock them) until they are straight or until parallel to the floor. Slowly return to starting position and repeat continuously. (Each lift = 1 count.)

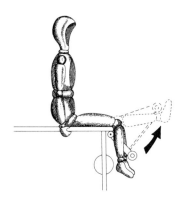

FIGURE 1.10 Quadriceps curl

RECORDING AND INTERPRETING YOUR SCORES

To understand the significance of your scores on the physical fitness tests, you may compare your scores with those made by others in the 17–25 age range and with the score you made on another test. For this purpose, Table I presents a set of "norms" with the scores converted to rankings based on the performance of a large number of other young adult men and women.

In Tables I and II, find your score and circle it for each test. Then look in the left-hand column to find your ranking. If you rank at Step V, you are better than 80 percent of college age people; if your score falls in the step IV category, you are better than 60 percent of the population sampled; a rating of Step III places you between the 40th and the 59th percentiles which is in the "average" range.

A score in the Step II range means you are below average and a Step I rating means you are in the lower 20 percent of the young adults sampled. Because the norms are based on college age students from a wide variety of backgrounds and fitness levels, being at Step II is probably an undesirable goal. You should strive to reach Step V ultimately, if you are in the 17–25 age range. Regardless of your score, the important thing to remember is that if

TABLE I.
Rankings for Test I–V*

Rank	minutes 1.5 mi. run/walk		inches sit & reach		crunch		repetitions push-up		pull-up	
	♂	♀	♂	♀	♂	♀	♂	♀	♂	♀
Step V	<10	<13	7>	8>	44>	34>	45>	30>	15>	3>
Step IV	11	14	4–6	6–7	39–43	31–33	38–44	26–29	11–14	2
Step III	12	15	1–3	2–5	35–38	28–30	32–37	21–25	7–10	1
Step II	13	16	-3– 2	2–1	30–34	25–27	26–31	14–20	4–6	25 sec.>
Step I	14>	17>	< 3	< 2	<29	<24	<25	<13	<3	<24 sec.

TABLE II.
Rankings for Tests VI–X*

	♂	♀
Step V	17>	15>
Step IV	12–16	11–14
Step III	9–11	8–10
Step II	5–8	4–7
Step I	<4	<3

*♂ norms for men; ♀ norms for women; norms for women include bent-arm hang time at steps I and II steps 1–2 and modified push-ups steps 1–5; < means "or less"; > means "or more".

you are already fit, you should strive to maintain it. If you are just beginning a program of fitness and your fitness is low, you should strive to improve over a period of time. Perhaps progressing one step every four weeks would be a reasonable goal for you. It takes time, so do not expect improvements overnight. Remember to record your scores on Charts I and II in the Appendix. At the end of the course, or at the end of three months, plot your scores on Tables I and II with a different colored pencil to observe your improvement.

SKINFOLD MEASURES

Measuring skinfolds requires someone familiar with the use of calipers. When done correctly by an expert, skinfold measures may be used to calculate body composition fairly accurately. The measurements are taken at four sites (the triceps, biceps, subscapula, and crest of the ilium) shown in Figure 1.11. The seven-step procedure is as follows: Using skinfold calipers such as the Lange or Lafayette, (1) locate the mid-point on the back of the right arm (triceps); lift the skinfold parallel to the long axis of the bone by pinching between the thumb and fingers, about 1/4 inch (1 cm.) above the site; hold the caliper parallel to the floor and allow the jaws to close. Hold for two seconds then read the dial to the nearest mm. Repeat the measurement until two successive readings have been made within one mm. of each other and record that score. Continue using this same technique and (2) measure a vertical skinfold over the mid-point of the front of the right arm (biceps); (3) measure a fold at the inferior angle of the right scapula (on a slight diagonal with the medial side being higher than the lateral); (4) measure at the crest of the ilium on the right side of the pelvis, directly below the armpit; this fold will be parallel with the floor or on a slight diagonal following the natural fold line. Now (5) add the scores of the four sites and use the total to find the percentage of body fat on Table III according to your age and gender. Finally (6) find your rank on Table IV and then (7) record your scores on Charts I and III in the Appendix.

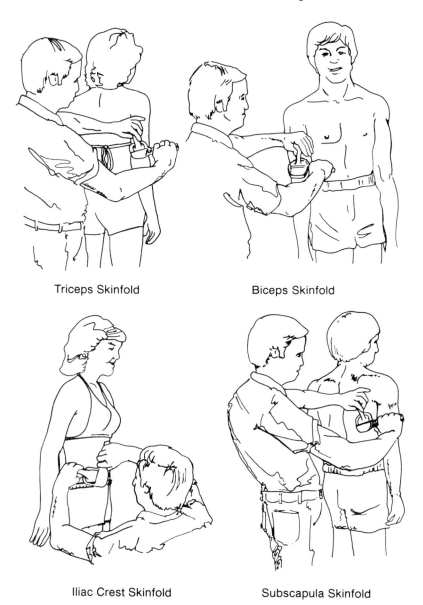

Triceps Skinfold   Biceps Skinfold

Iliac Crest Skinfold   Subscapula Skinfold

FIGURE 1.11 Four skinfold sites

TABLE III*
Estimated Percent of Body Fat
(from sum of biceps, triceps, scapular, and iliac skinfolds)

Sum of 4 Skinfolds (mm)	Males (age in years)				Females (age in years)			
	17–29	30–39	40–49	50+	16–29	30–39	40–49	50+
15	4.8	—	—	—	10.5	—	—	—
20	8.1	12.2	12.2	12.6	14.1	17.0	19.8	21.4
25	10.5	14.2	15.0	15.6	16.8	19.4	22.2	24.0
30	12.9	16.2	17.7	18.6	19.5	21.8	24.5	26.6
35	14.7	17.7	19.6	20.8	21.5	23.7	26.4	28.5
40	16.4	19.2	21.4	22.9	23.4	25.5	28.2	30.3
45	17.7	20.4	23.0	24.7	25.0	26.9	29.6	31.9
50	19.0	21.5	24.6	26.5	26.5	28.2	31.0	33.4
55	20.1	22.5	25.9	27.9	27.8	29.4	32.1	34.6
60	21.2	23.5	27.1	29.2	29.1	30.6	33.2	35.7
65	22.2	24.3	28.2	30.4	30.2	31.6	34.1	36.7
70	23.1	25.1	29.3	31.6	31.2	32.5	35.0	37.7
75	24.0	25.9	30.3	32.7	32.2	33.4	35.9	38.7
80	24.8	26.6	31.2	33.8	33.1	34.3	36.7	39.6
85	25.5	27.2	32.1	34.8	34.0	35.1	37.5	40.4
90	26.2	27.8	33.0	35.8	34.8	35.8	38.3	41.2
95	26.9	28.4	33.7	36.6	35.6	36.5	39.0	41.9
100	27.6	29.0	34.4	37.4	36.4	37.2	39.7	42.6
105	28.2	29.6	35.1	38.2	37.1	37.9	40.4	43.3
110	28.8	30.1	35.8	39.0	37.8	38.6	41.0	43.9
115	29.4	30.6	36.4	39.7	38.4	39.1	41.5	44.5
120	30.0	31.1	37.0	40.4	39.0	39.6	42.0	45.1
125	30.5	31.5	37.6	41.1	39.6	40.1	42.5	45.7
130	31.0	31.9	38.2	41.8	40.2	40.6	43.0	46.2
135	31.5	32.3	38.7	42.4	40.8	41.1	43.5	46.7
140	32.0	32.7	39.2	43.0	41.3	41.6	44.0	47.2
145	32.5	33.1	39.7	43.6	41.8	42.1	44.5	47.7
150	32.9	33.5	40.2	44.1	42.3	42.6	45.0	48.2
155	33.3	33.9	40.7	44.6	42.8	43.1	45.4	48.7
160	33.7	34.3	41.2	45.1	43.3	43.6	45.8	49.2
165	34.1	34.6	41.6	45.6	43.7	44.0	46.2	49.6
170	34.5	34.8	42.0	46.1	44.1	44.4	46.6	50.0
175	34.9	—	—	—	—	44.8	47.0	50.4
180	35.3	—	—	—	—	45.2	47.4	50.8
185	35.6	—	—	—	—	45.6	47.8	51.2
190	35.9	—	—	—	—	45.9	48.2	51.6
195	—	—	—	—	—	46.2	48.5	52.0
200	—	—	—	—	—	46.5	48.8	52.4
205	—	—	—	—	—	—	49.1	52.7
210	—	—	—	—	—	—	49.4	53.0

In two-thirds of the instances the error was within ±3.5% of the bodyweight as fat for the women and ±5% for the men.

*Adapted with permission from: "Body Fat Assessed from Total Body Density" and its Estimation From Skinfold Thickness by J. V. G. A. Durnin and J. Womersley, *British Journal of Nutrition,* Volume 32, Page 95, 1974, Cambridge University Press, New York City, New York.

TABLE IV
Body Composition Norms (Ages 18–60)

Rank	Men % of Fat	Women % of Fat
Obese	25 >	30 >
Optimal Health	10–24	18–29
Optimal Fitness	17–18	16–25
Most Athletes	5–13	12–22
Minimal	5–10	15–18

HEIGHT AND WEIGHT

Height-Weight Tables are widely used. These are based on average weights of hundreds of individuals of the same height, age, and frame size. The population on which these tables are based does not necessarily represent the general population of the United States, nor do the tables consider the relative amount of fat content; therefore, they should not be considered as totally accurate. To use Table VI, it is necessary to determine your frame size. Wrist circumference is a helpful but not totally accurate predictor of the size of one's skeleton. Have a partner measure the wrist by placing the tape above the styloid processes (wrist bones) at the smallest circumference. Record it on Chart I (Appendix) then refer to Table V to find your approximate skeletal (frame) size. Your height should be measured on a stadiometer. Record this on Chart I, also.

TABLE V
Frame Size Based on Wrist Circumference

	Men	Women
Small Frame	6½″ or less	5½″ or less
Medium Frame	6¾″–7¼″	5¾″
Large Frame	7½″ or more	6″ or more

TABLE VI
1983 Metropolitan Height and Weight Tables for Men and Women
According to Frame, Ages 25–59

Height (In Shoes)†		Weight in Pounds (In Indoor Clothing)*		
		Small Frame	Medium Frame	Large Frame
Feet	Inches		**Men**	
5	2	128–134	131–141	138–150
5	3	130–136	133–143	140–153
5	4	132–138	135–145	142–156
5	5	134–140	137–148	144–160
5	6	136–142	139–151	146–164
5	7	138–145	142–154	149–168
5	8	140–148	145–157	152–172
5	9	142–151	148–160	155–176
5	10	144–154	151–163	158–180
5	11	146–157	154–166	161–184
6	0	149–160	157–170	164–188
6	1	152–164	160–174	168–192
6	2	155–168	164–178	172–197
6	3	158–172	167–182	176–202
6	4	162–176	171–187	181–207
			Women	
4	10	102–111	109–121	118–131
4	11	103–113	111–123	120–134
5	0	104–115	113–126	122–137
5	1	106–118	115–129	125–140
5	2	108–121	118–132	128–143
5	3	111–124	121–135	131–147
5	4	114–127	124–138	134–151
5	5	117–130	127–141	137–155
5	6	120–133	130–144	140–159
5	7	123–136	133–147	143–163
5	8	126–139	136–150	146–167
5	9	129–142	139–153	149–170
5	10	132–145	142–156	152–173
5	11	135–148	145–159	155–176
6	0	138–151	148–162	158–179

*Indoor clothing weighing 5 pounds for men and 3 pounds for women.
†Shoes with 1-inch heels.
Courtesy of Statistical Bulletin of Metropolitan Life Insurance Company

Notice that the height on the chart assumes you are wearing 1-inch heels. If your actual height was measured in stocking-feet at, for example, 5'7", then you should add an inch and use 5'8" on Table VI to find your optimum weight. *Notice* also that the Table was developed for men and women ages 25–59. Therefore, if you are between the ages of 18 and 25, you should subtract one pound for each year under 25. *Notice* finally, that the Table allows for five pounds of clothing (including shoes) for men and three pounds of clothing (including shoes) for women. If you are weighing in a leotard or gym suit, you will weigh one or two pounds lighter than you would in "street clothes." If you weigh barefooted, you will weigh a pound or two less than the chart allows for. To read Table VI, find your height (with shoes) in the left column of the Table which is appropriate to your sex; then, with a straight-edge, read directly across to the column which is appropriate for your frame size. Record your "ideal weight" range on Chart I in the Appendix.

BODY MASS INDEX

To determine your Body Mass Index (BMI), use the following formula: BMI = (Weight in kg) divided by (Height in cm)^2. These calculations have been made for you on the nomogram in Figure 1.12. All weights and heights in the nomogram are *without* shoes or clothing. If you have weighed and measured *with clothing,* then to allow for shoes and clothing, men should add five pounds and women should add three pounds. One inch in height should be added for shoes for both men and women. To read the nomogram, place a straight-edge across the scale between your height (the column on the left) and your weight (right hand column). Then read the scale in the middle where the straight-edge intersects it. This will give you your BMI and your weight ranking. The latter will tell you whether you are at (a) a desirable weight, (b) 20 percent overweight or (c) 40 percent overweight. Women should use the rankings on the left side of the center scale and men should use the rankings on the right side of the center scale. Table VII below gives the norms for your BMI. Record your scores on Chart III in the Appendix.

TABLE VII. BMI Norms for Ages 16>		
Rank	♀	♂
Desirable	<22	<22
Average	24.7	23.5
Obese	27.2	26.9
Morbidly Obese	31.8	31.4

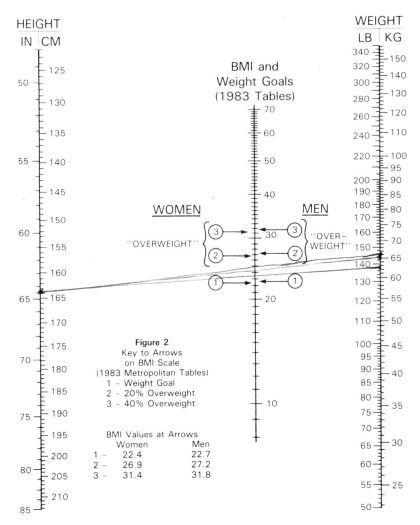

The ratio weight/height² (metric units) is read from the central scale after a straight edge is placed between height and body weight.

FIGURE 1.12 Nomogram for body mass index (kg/m²) (1983 Metropolitan Life Insurance Co. tables [2]). Weights and heights are without clothing. With clothes, add 5 lb (2.3 kg) for men or 3 lb for women, and 1 in. (2.5 cm) in height for shoes.

Courtesy, Statistical Bulletin, Metropolitan Life Insurance Company.

RELATIVE WEIGHT

Another simple estimate for characterizing one's degree of obesity or leanness is *Relative Weight* (RW). This simple calculation provides a single number or index indicating percentage of desirable weight. RW = actual body weight (with shoes and clothes) divided by the medium frame desirable weight for your height. To find the latter, refer to Table VI and find your height and then read across to the medium frame column which gives a range of desirable weights for that height. Now determine the mid-point of that range by adding the lowest and highest numbers and dividing by two. When you have determined the mid-point for a medium frame person of your height, then divide it into your actual weight to determine your RW, i.e., the percentage you are over or underweight. (For example, a 5'7" woman weighs 150 pounds. Table VI lists 133–147 as a desirable weight range for a medium frame. The average for a medium frame is thus, 147 + 133 = 280 ÷ 2 = 140. RW = 150 ÷ 140 = 1.07. The woman is 107 percent of her desirable weight or 7 percent overweight.) Record your actual weight on Chart III in the Appendix and record your RW on the same chart.

WAIST/HIP GIRTH RATIO

The last indicator of your fat/lean status to be calculated is the ratio between your waist and hip girth. Have someone measure your waist and hips with a tape measure. The waist (W)/hip (H) ratio should then be calculated as follows: W:H = waist girth ÷ by hip girth. (For example, in a man having a waist girth of 30 inches and a hip girth of 32, W:H = 30 ÷ 32 = .93.) In women the desirable ratio is .8 or less and in men the desirable ratio is 1.0 or less. Record your ratio on Chart III in the Appendix.

The significance of these measures of Skinfold (Percentage Fat), Weight, Body Mass Index, Relative Weight, and Waist/Hip Girth Ratio are discussed in chapter 6. As explained previously, the purpose of using several measures is to compensate for the lack of reliability of any one measure by looking for trends among several. By looking at the results of all of these, you should have a reasonably good assessment of your body composition.

"IDEAL" MEASUREMENTS

It is difficult to define what we mean by "ideal" measurements when referring to the figure/physique. At one time in history, Venus De Milo, with her 43" bust, 38" waist and 44" hips, was considered the perfect female figure. Very few women today feel that these measurements are ideal; neither do most men accept the 18" neck, 54" chest and 19" arm of a "Mr. Universe" as a perfect physique for them. Fashions and fads have much to do with what we consider ideal.

Body build influences your measurements. A person with a large bony structure naturally has larger measurements than a person with small bones, yet each measurement can be considered ideal for that individual. There are three basic types of body builds that we may inherit. These are classified according to linearity, muscularity, and fat distribution. The *ectomorph* is slender, characterized by having a large forehead, small bones, a long, slender neck, slender arms and legs, a narrow chest, round shoulders with winged scapulae, a flat abdomen, and inconspicuous buttocks. The *mesomorph* has firm muscles and large bones, and is ruggedly built with prominent facial bones, a rather long, muscular neck, wide, sloping shoulders, a broad chest, muscular arms, a heavily muscled abdomen, a low waist, narrow hips, muscular buttocks, and powerful legs. The *endomorph* is round and soft and characterized by having a round head, a short neck, narrow shoulders, fatty breasts and abdomen, short arms, wide hips, heavy buttocks, and short, heavy legs. Few people have a build which perfectly fits one of these types. More than likely you are a combination type, such as an ecto-mesomorph or a meso-endomorph.

Because of hereditary differences in our body build, it is not realistic to expect the majority of the population to have the same body proportions. However, because of a national preoccupation with body measurements, the following guidelines are offered, based on the measurements of thousands of men and women who are considered well proportioned.

TABLE VIII
Body Proportion Guidelines*

	Men	Women
Chest/Bust	Same as hip	(see hip)
Waist	5–7″ less than chest or hip	8–10″ smaller than bust
Abdomen	1½–2½″ smaller than chest	1½–2½″ smaller than bust
Hips	Same as chest	same as bust if slim hips 1–3″ larger than bust for av. hips 3–4″ larger than bust for full hips
Thighs	8–10″ less than waist	6–7″ less than waist
Calves	7–8″ less than thigh	6–7″ less than thigh
Ankles	6–7″ less than calves	5–6″ less than calves
Upper Arm	Twice the circumference of the wrist	twice the circumference of the wrist

*From *The West Point Fitness and Diet Book,* by Colonel James L. Anderson and Martin Cohen, Copyright © 1977 by Colonel James L. Anderson and Martin Cohen. Reprinted by permission of Rawson, Wade Publishers.

HOW TO MEASURE

Record your measurements on Charts I and II in the Appendix, along with the goals you are striving to achieve. Measurements should be taken by a partner because you cannot measure yourself accurately. Stand relaxed with your weight evenly distributed on both feet, arms at sides. Do not suck-in your waist or contract muscles to alter your measurements. The tape measure should be kept parallel to the floor and pulled snugly but not tight enough to indent the skin. You should wear as little clothing as possible (underwear, bathing suit or leotards), and when you are measured at later dates, make certain that you are dressed in the same manner. It is also advisable always to measure at the same time of day if an accurate record of progress is to be kept. Do not measure after exercise, since the muscles will be temporarily enlarged. Measure to the nearest eighth-of-an-inch (or centimeter if the metric scale is used).

Bust—Partner should stand and measure from the front at the largest girth (nipple line) at the mid-point of a normal breath.

Waist—Partner should stand and measure from the front at the smallest girth between the ribs and the crest of the ilium.

Abdomen—Partner should kneel and measure from the side at the largest girth between waist and hips, usually just below the navel.

Hips—Partner should kneel and measure from the side at the largest girth, approximately level with the pubic bone.

Thigh—Partner should kneel in front and measure upper thigh of the dominant leg* at the largest girth, usually an inch or two below the crotch and directly under buttocks.

Calf—Partner should kneel at the side and measure the largest girth of the dominant leg* usually about two-thirds of the way up from the ankle.

Ankle—Partner should kneel at the side and measure the smallest girth of the dominant leg just above the ankle bones.

Upper Arm—Partner should stand at the side and measure over the largest part of the bicep, midway between the shoulder and elbow. The subject should raise the dominant arm, face the palm up parallel to floor, and relax the arm. The tape should be perpendicular to the floor.

REFERENCES

1. Chisolm, D. M. et al. *Par-Q Validation Report,* British Columbia Ministry of Health, Victoria, B.C., May 1978.
2. Lamb, L. "The Dangerous Pot," *The Health Letter,* 25:10(1985).
3. Wilmore, J. H. et al. "Body Composition: A Round Table," *The Physician and Sports Medicine* 14:3 (March 1986):146–162.

*Dominant leg is the leg you would normally use to kick a ball.

Fitness

2

PRETEST

1. What constitutes total fitness?
2. What is physical fitness?
3. Why is it so important for you to exercise regularly?
4. What happens to your body while you are exercising vigorously?
5. What happens to your body after you have exercised regularly for a period of weeks?

In the last half of the twentieth century, interest in the physical aspects of good health (wellness) has grown rapidly, and it shows no signs of waning. Leading national organizations such as the American Alliance for Health, Physical Education, Recreation and Dance; the American Heart Association; the American Medical Association; the President's Council on Physical Fitness and Sport; and the Public Health Service encourage and support the principle that individuals should have a healthy life style and be physically fit. Each day millions of feet travel the jogging trails or push the pedals of a bicycle while innumerable individuals "work up a sweat" on the racquetball courts, soccer fields, and gymnasium floors. Many choose to be active for the joy of it; others, having accepted the premise that being physically active can provide all kinds of benefits, do it for the health of it.

Being physically active to become physically fit is only one of the basic ingredients of total fitness. Exercise should be combined with proper diet, rest and relaxation, abstention from tobacco usage, abstention from or moderation in alcohol usage, and wise management of stress to add years to your life (quantity) and life to your years (quality).

POSITIVE HEALTH CONCEPTS

Good health is a possession to be valued highly, but most individuals are not concerned with maintaining or improving it until it is seriously threatened. It is something you cannot buy in a drugstore or health food store, nor can it be given to you. You have to work to achieve this aspect of the "good life;" you have to do it yourself. The positive qualities to strive for are:

1. A high energy level developed through improved physical fitness, particularly of the cardiovascular and respiratory systems (achieved by exercising vigorously).
2. Optimal muscle strength, endurance, and mobility (achieved by exercising vigorously).
3. Optimal nutrition (achieved by consuming the right foods in the right amounts).
4. An ideal body composition—a lean body with a low percentage of fat (achieved by observing nos. 1, 2, and 3 above).
5. The ability to relax and sleep (aided by a vigorous life style, regular habits of rest, and the use of relaxation techniques).
6. A happy disposition and excellent mental health (achieved through continuing emotional growth).
7. A well integrated personality (resulting from the first 6).[1]

The extent to which you develop your health potential depends upon your life style. It is worth the effort to make changes in your living patterns in order to develop these positive health qualities. Being "healthy" means that you can get through the stresses of the day and still have the energy to meet unexpected demands and the desire to be active in leisure pursuits. It can be the difference between attending or cutting classes, working or missing a pay check, being safe or having an accident, being comfortable or aching, enjoying or loathing an activity. With good health you will be able to live more effectively within your capabilities—now is the time to begin to improve your life style.

PHYSICAL FITNESS DEFINED

Physical fitness, a quality of positive health, is specific to each individual. It is the "physical condition" that allows you to do your work efficiently and effectively, pursue leisure time activities vigorously and alertly, and respond to physical emergencies successfully during an ordinary day. There is a difference of opinion as to what components constitute physical fitness, because some authors list only health-related components while others expand the list to include skill-related factors such as agility, power, speed, balance, reaction time, and coordination. Skill-related fitness is important, but this text limits discussion to the five basic components of health-related fitness—strength, muscular endurance, cardiovascular endurance, flexibility, and body composition.

Strength is measured by the amount of force a muscle, or group of muscles, can exert against resistance in a single maximum effort. For example, if you can lift a greater weight than someone else in a single lift, you are said to be stronger than that person.

Muscular endurance may be defined as the ability of a muscle, or group of muscles, to apply force repeatedly or to sustain a contraction for a long period of time. For example, performing "crunches" for 60 seconds tests the dynamic endurance of the hip and abdominal muscles, and performing the bent arm hang for 10 seconds tests the static endurance of the arm and shoulder muscles.

Cardiovascular endurance (sometimes referred to as cardiorespiratory endurance) is a measure of the ability of the heart and lungs to provide fuel to the tissues and carry off waste products during sustained exercise. It is commonly referred to as one's "wind." A typical test of this type of endurance is to run for as long as possible. The sooner you become winded and the longer it takes you to recover "your breath" and resting heart rate, the poorer your cardiovascular endurance.

Flexibility is a measure of the range of motion in the joints of the body. The length of the muscles, tendons, and ligaments largely determines how much freedom of motion one has. Stretching exercises are used to increase flexibility. For example, your ability to assume a long-sitting position and touch your toes without bending your knees is a measure of the flexibility in your lower back and posterior leg muscles.

Body composition is the relative percentage of fat and lean (fat free) body mass. Percentage of body fat is measured by several different methods; a simple method is measuring the thickness of subcutaneous fat and a complex one is using the underwater weighing technique.

WHY EXERCISE?

As we enter the last decade of the twentieth century, the age of technology has given way to the age of information. Automation continues to escalate and the number of jobs that require little, if any, physical effort continues to increase. As your need for physical activity does not decrease, it then becomes imperative for you to make exercise an integral part of your normal life style. "If you do not use it, you will lose it!"

Organically, humans are active creatures—you are not meant to lead a sedentary life. You possess the capacities for movement and the neuromuscular mechanism to produce it, and your growth and development depend upon physical activity. According to the "law of use and disuse," without activity, atrophy (wasting away) of size and function sets in and experiences become limited.

Your body has 206 bones and 639 muscles. The muscles are made up of uncounted millions of muscle fibers. Each fiber possesses a slender nerve strand which fires up to 75 impulses per second. There are thousands of miles of nerves and thousands of nerve centers which determine your movements, thoughts, memories, and imagination. Your heart pumps 13 tons of blood per day (you have 5 to 6 quarts of blood) through 100,000 miles of blood vessels. To keep this complex mechanism in working order, exercise, which contributes to total fitness, is essential.

While you are in school, it is usually easy to find time and space to exercise, since the facilities and opportunities are available. After graduation, many people stop exercising regularly because "workout" areas and equipment are not as accessible, interests change, while demands of job and home crowd out recreational pursuits. As a result, the adult must make an extra effort to keep exercise in the daily routine, since the need continues throughout life. Therefore, plan and prepare now to make wise use of your leisure time today, tomorrow, and in years to come.

If you choose to not be physically active, you may be looking forward to having a body that is not pleasing to the eye and does not perform efficiently. Lack of exercise, combined with growing older, can cause a multitude of negative results including:

1. Decreased flexibility—You may be "stiff in the joints!"
2. Decreased body leanness—You may be fat!
3. Loss of bone density—You may develop osteoporosis!
4. Decreased muscle strength—You may develop a variety of aches and pains!
5. Decreased cardiovascular fitness level—You cannot run and play and work with ease!
6. Decreased circulatory efficiency—you may die at a rather young age!

IMMEDIATE EFFECTS OF EXERCISE

The effects of physical activity upon the tissues and functions of the body depend upon a number of factors including the type of exercise, the intensity and length of the workout, and your training state.

Very light exercise, continued for a short period of time, produces negligible effect upon the body. Fairly strenuous activity, continued for a reasonable period of time, has certain immediate physiological effects on the body. These may be stated briefly as follows:

1. Cardiac output increases as a result of increased heart rate and stroke volume. The effect of the increased blood supply is to bring greater amounts of food and oxygen to body cells and to carry away waste products of cellular activity more rapidly.
2. Oxygen uptake is increased as the breathing rate becomes more frequent and inhalation deepens. This change is necessary in order to supply the greater amount of oxygen to the working muscles and to remove waste products.
3. Heat loss increases as the elimination system works to keep the body temperature at 39° C, primarily by evaporation (sweating).
4. Metabolic rate increases during the exercise, and for several hours afterwards, as more calories are burned to supply necessary energy.
5. Working muscles increase in volume due to the increased blood flow.
6. Blood flow to strategic areas (working muscles, heart, skin, adipose tissue, and lungs) increases while the flow to less active areas (kidneys, liver, stomach, and intestines) decreases to ensure an adequate supply of oxygen and to remove waste products.
7. Systolic and diastolic pressures rise during static contractions and when small groups of muscles (such as in the arms) are used above waist level to help force blood to the working muscles.
8. Systolic pressure rises during dynamic exercises, primarily because of increased cardiac output.
9. Skin becomes red as the blood flow to the surface increases to carry away excessive heat.
10. Body cells are stimulated through the increased blood and lymph supplies.

When one engages regularly in a moderate amount of invigorating physical activity, the mechanisms of respiration, circulation, and elimination become increasingly more efficient in their functions of supplying food and oxygen to working cells and eliminating waste products. Regular exercise of reasonable intensity and duration, then, vitalizes and invigorates the body tissues, raising their efficiency to a higher level. Lack of exercise tends to cause tissues to become inefficient in performing their functions.

LONG RANGE HEALTH BENEFITS OF REGULAR EXERCISE

Most medical and health leaders agree that regular exercise should be an important part of your lifestyle. The benefits received from training will vary among individuals; they are dependent upon your age, current fitness level, and type of exercise as well as the frequency, intensity, and duration (time) of the workout. Research has shown that training will produce many positive results; some that will be of primary interest to you are included here:

1. The aging process is delayed as you operate at a much higher level of efficiency—your "body parts" work much better.
2. Life expectancy increases as your chances of having it cut short by various illnesses and conditions decrease.
3. Training has been found to decrease the probability of:
   a. Angina
   b. Arteriosclerosis
   c. Asthma
   d. Backache
   e. Chronic heart disease
   f. Chronic lung disease
   g. Hypertension
   h. Diabetes mellitus
   i. Obesity
   j. Osteoporosis
4. Survival rate from a coronary disease rises and recovery rate from other diseases and debilitating conditions is likely to be faster.
5. Minor aches and pains, stiffness, and soreness appear less frequently.
6. Tension is reduced and ability to relax improves.
7. Chronic fatigue occurs less often.
8. Injury rate and severity of an injury decreases.
9. Physical fitness level improves as you increase your strength, muscular endurance, cardiovascular endurance, flexibility, and body leanness.
10. General appearance improves.

ANATOMICAL AND PHYSIOLOGICAL CHANGES

The benefits listed previously are in large part due to several anatomical and physiological changes which accompany improvement in strength, muscular endurance, cardiovascular endurance, flexibility, and leanness. These are summarized as follows:

1. The aerobic capacity (maximum oxygen uptake), cardiac output, and stroke volume increase. As a result, your resting heart rate will be lower and there will be a smaller increase in heart rate for a given increase in work. (cardiovascular endurance training)
2. The blood volume increases which allows the needs of the circulatory and elimination systems to be met more efficiently. (cardiovascular and muscular/endurance training)
3. The number of working capillaries increases resulting in improved vascularization. This is particularly important for coronary collateral circulation. (cardiovascular and muscle endurance training)
4. Muscular strength and endurance improves and chronic hypertrophy results from an increase in the size of existing muscle fibers. (body composition training)

5. Neuromuscular efficiency increases because of:
    a. the reduction of fatty tissues in the muscles.
    b. the decreased resistance from opposing muscles.
    c. more efficient transmission of nerve impulses.
    d. less wasted motion.
    e. improved efficiency in the contractile processes of the muscle fibers.
6. Joint cartilages become thicker and tendons and ligaments become larger and stronger.
7. Bones increase in density, especially with weight bearing exercise.
8. Interior lung volume increases, allowing a larger exchange of air per breath. This results in a decreased respiratory rate during rest and a smaller increase in breathing rate during heavy workouts.

REFERENCES

1. H. A. DeVries, *Health Science: A Positive Approach* (Santa Monica, Ca.: Goodyear Publishing Company, Inc., 1979).

Beginning Your Exercise Program

3

PRETEST

1. What are important points to know before you begin an exercise program?
2. What are basic rules to follow when participating in a workout?
3. How do you select exercises to meet specific needs?
4. Why are some exercises to be used with caution, if at all?
5. How long will it take you to reach an adequate level of physical fitness?
6. What are factors to consider when setting up a training program?

Exercises are not a panacea but regular participation in a well planned exercise program is a major health plus. Fitness must be a vital part of your lifestyle, not an "on-again and off-again" experience if you expect to receive and keep the benefits. The information in this chapter is to assist you in selecting the type and the amount of activity necessary to develop and/or to maintain your desired or acceptable level of fitness, and to improve your health status and personal appearance.

POINTS TO CONSIDER BEFORE BEGINNING YOUR EXERCISE PROGRAM

To receive the "pluses and not the minuses" from an exercise program you should be knowledgeable about many factors. Prior to beginning you should:

1. Take a good look at yourself and assess your current level of fitness and state of mind. (See chapter 1.)
2. Determine your goals and objectives. Why are you beginning an exercise program? What do you expect to gain?
3. Be realistic. Do not expect changes overnight; you did not get into your present shape quickly.

4. Have a thorough medical examination and the approval of your physician before you participate, if you have been leading a sedentary lifestyle. Seek the advice of your physician if you have an illness, operation, or injury after you have begun your exercise program. (See Par-Q test on p. 1)

5. Be knowledgeable about "how to" select the correct exercises/physical activities and "how to" properly perform them. Be aware of the inherent hazards in some physical activities such as rowing, jogging, and weight training.

6. Remember that exercise combined with reduction in caloric intake is by far the most satisfactory method of losing weight.

7. Fit the regimen into your schedule. The time of day is not important except you should avoid working out right after a meal (wait at least two hours).

8. Take note of the weather conditions. Generally, it is not wise to work out of doors when it is hot and humid, cold and windy, or smoggy.

9. Remember that firm muscles are more attractive than sagging ones. If you are a female, you should not be concerned with developing bulging muscles as it is highly improbable that you will do so.

10. Know that extensive exercise may decrease your appetite. Even if it does not, studies show that any increase is negligible and that you will burn more calories than you take in.

11. Avoid taking measurements immediately after exercise because muscles tend to hypertrophy (increase in size) during and immediately after exercise.

12. Expect your bone structure to stay the same. After childhood, the primary effect of weight bearing exercise on the skeletal system is to increase bone density rather than volume.

13. Remember that heredity is a major factor in determining appearance. Exercising makes it easier for you to attain and maintain a desired shape and size but will not solve all posture and figure/physique problems.

14. Continue with a regular program of activity to maintain the training effect. You will return to your pretraining level of fitness very quickly if you stop exercising.

15. Be aware that you could suffer an injury. Endurance activities which require running and jumping generally cause more debilitating injuries to beginning exercisers than non-weight bearing activities.

16. Women, be active during your menstrual periods. Lack of proper exercise is often a cause of dysmenorrhea. (See chapter 12.)

17. Women, be aware that those who train extensively and have a very low percentage of body fat may have secondary amenorrhea (stop menstruating). For many, this results in a loss of bone density and vital minerals, particularly iron.

18. Be active as there is no such thing as "effortless exercise." Fancy machines, girdles, belts, and couches are not effective for "spot reducing," "breaking up cellulite," or "melting away fat"—they shrink only your bank account!

GENERAL SUGGESTIONS FOR EXERCISING

In order to gain the maximum benefit and enjoyment from an exercise program (for conditioning and/or reducing), and at the same time to suffer a minimum of discomfort, you will find the following suggestions useful.

1. Wear comfortable, lightweight, breathable clothing so that you can move freely and safely. A cotton top and cotton shorts are very good choices because cotton allows sweat to evaporate easily. Women wear bras; men wear athletic supporters.
2. Wear good supportive shoes that are suitable for the activity.
3. Plan a definite time for your workouts and adhere to it—preferably the same time each day. Make it as vital a part of your daily routine as bathing and dressing!
4. Exercise early or late in the day if the weather is hot and humid; a temperature of 70° F with 85 percent humidity is considered to be the beginning of the danger zone. Acclimate your body to the higher temperature by exercising 10 to 15 minutes the first day and gradually moving into your normal routine.
5. Know your target heart rate range and work within it. (See page 43.)
6. Keep the exercise period relatively short (20 to 40 minutes) and well organized to avoid boredom, discouragement, and injury. Strength and muscular endurance exercises might be performed on Mondays, Wednesdays, and Fridays, and cardiovascular endurance activities on Tuesdays, Thursdays, and Saturdays. Flexibility exercises should be included with every workout.
7. Start each workout with a warm-up; this part of each workout should include low-intensity aerobic exercise to warm up the heart muscles and stretching exercises. Special attention should be given to flexibility; do slow static stretching.
8. Find a comfortable position to begin an exercise, and stabilize other body parts to prevent muscle strain. Use padding to avoid pressure on bony areas which might become bruised and tender.
9. Start the exercise (one that is in your ability range) with a minimum number of repetitions and increase the number gradually over a period of time (progressive overload) until you reach your goal.
10. Do not over do it. You should not be sore and stiff the next day. Know your level of ability and do not attempt to keep pace with your peers. Work at your level, not theirs.
11. Be aware of signs of overexertion and stop if you:
    a. Feel nauseous.
    b. Cannot talk normally and have difficulty breathing.
    c. Become dizzy or lightheaded.
    d. Begin to shake.
    e. Experience chest, arm, or facial pain or tightness in the chest.
    f. Have a very pale or flushed face.

    g. Begin to perspire excessively.

    h. Feel exceptionally weak and/or lose muscle control.

12. Keep emergency medication for chronic conditions (such as for diabetes or asthma) with you and notify someone (preferably the instructor) of your condition.

13. Be careful when performing aerobic workouts with hand held weights. The maximum weight should be three pounds but begin with one-half pound weights. Avoid using ankle weights as they can cause stress fractures and achilles tendinitis.

14. Breathe normally during the performance of the exercise. If you will exhale on the effort phase (lifting your body weight in a push-up or a free weight) and inhale during the recovery phase (lowering your body weight or a free weight), the exercise may seem easier. Do not hold your breath!

15. Perform exercises slowly (no quick, jerky motions) to help prevent soreness and injury. Emphasize proper technique and full range of motion. Exercise slowly and rhythmically, concentrating on strong muscular effort.

16. Exercise the entire body. Do not spend the entire workout concentrating on one set of muscles alone. Pay attention to the weak areas and do not perform only the exercise that you like.

17. Maintain the fun element; you should leave the workout refreshed in body and in mind. If it becomes a drudgery, add a variety of exercises, companionship, music, or new scenery.

18. Drink plenty of liquids; plain water is an excellent fluid replacement. Do not rely on your thirst mechanism as it may not indicate a need for fluids. Drinking a pint of water 30 minutes prior to exercise time should prepare your body adequately. Then, if the workout is long (40 minutes or more), drink about one-half a cup of water approximately every 15 minutes.

19. End each workout with a cool-down to ease your body back into its normal state. Slow, gentle stretches are effective along with slow walking after an intense workout. A warm shower will complete that feeling of "relaxed well-being."

EXERCISES FOR FIGURE/PHYSIQUE IMPROVEMENT

Physical fitness, posture, figure/physique, and weight control are interrelated and overlapping. The same exercises can be used for all these purposes. And, believe it or not, the same exercise which helps the flabby person *decrease* measurements may help the thin person *increase* measurements.

    Both localized exercises (those for specific areas such as push-ups for the upper trunk and arms), and general exercises (such as jogging and swimming) are effective in "taking off inches." We suggest you do both to ensure that all muscle groups receive maximum benefit. Also, we strongly urge you to participate in dance and sports; their psychological value will complement their sociological and physiological benefits.

When designing a program to "shape-up," choose specific calisthenics for selected body regions you want to improve. Generally, it will be to your advantage to combine these with weight training and aerobic exercises. Both men and women can benefit from weight training exercises if they desire changes in their shapes. For some, calisthenics might not produce sufficient overload to bring about strengthening with accompanying muscle definition. Most women and many men cannot develop pronounced muscle definition because of genetic factors, but, generally, males, because of the presence of the hormone testosterone and greater muscle mass will have a greater degree of muscle hypertrophy than females.

Finally, remember that weight and figure/physique are not synonymous. If you consider yourself too broad in the hips or fat around the middle, this doesn't necessarily mean that you need to lose weight. If your weight approaches normalcy, your problem may be flabbiness or fat—not weight.

QUESTIONABLE EXERCISES

Not all exercises are good nor are all good exercises beneficial for all. You must become consumer-wise because everything that is touted to promote health and well-being will not be effective. Many popular magazines, television shows, and self-proclaimed health authorities advocate exercises which are harmful, as well as ineffective. The following are examples of commonly used exercises and some cautions to be observed.

Questionable Abdominal Exercises

Double Leg Lifts. Raising and lowering straight legs from a back-lying position is a dangerous exercise because it puts great strain on the lower back and may stretch or even rupture the abdominal muscles. This is not an abdominal-strengthening exercise, because the abdominal muscles are not attached to the legs. The muscles used are the hip flexors. If you had strong enough abdominal muscles to keep your back from arching during this exercise, it probably would not be harmful—but then, you would not need the exercise.

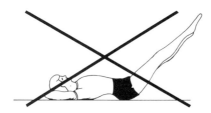

FIGURE 3.1 Double leg lifts

Sit-ups with Legs Straight. Like the double leg lift, this sit-up exercise uses the hip flexor muscles rather than the abdominals and may result in the same undesirable arched back and stretched abdominals. If it is executed so that the pelvis is tilted backward, and the lower back remains in contact with the floor while the spine curls up, it probably will not be harmful.

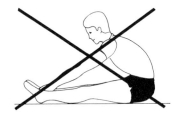

FIGURE 3.2 Sit-ups with legs straight

Sit-ups or Crunches with Hands Behind the Neck. Placing your hands in this position creates a pull on the neck and tends to place pressure on the cervical spine, and promotes a forward head posture. To avoid this potential problem, place the hands on your ears or fold your arms across your chest.

The safest, most effective abdominal strengthening exercises are trunk curls (crunches, see page 4) or isometric exercises. When adequate strength has been developed, sit-ups with bent knees might be attempted—but remember to curl up and keep your lower back flat. More advanced curls can be done by changing the arm position, using a tilt board, or adding weights.

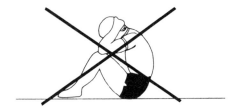

FIGURE 3.3 Sit-ups with hands behind the neck

Questionable Back Exercises

Lumbar Hyperextension. If you have lordosis (swayback), weak abdominals, or back problems, you should avoid exercises which allow the pelvis to tilt forward to stretch the abdominal muscles or arch (concave position) the back. Such exercises as back bends, prone arm and leg lifts (swan position), backward circling of the trunk, prone head and leg lifts, and push-ups if the abdominal muscles are not strong enough to keep the body from sagging are not recommended.

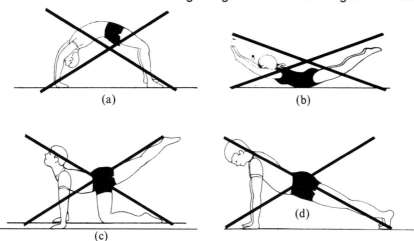

FIGURE 3.4 (a) Incorrect back bends. (b) Incorrect prone arm and leg lifts. (c) Incorrect kneeling head and leg lifts. (d) Incorrect push-ups.

Questionable Neck Exercises

Cervical Hyperextension. Doing neck hyperextensions can pinch arteries and nerves at the base of the skull (cervical spine area).

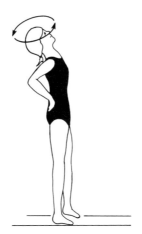

FIGURE 3.5 Neck circles

Neck Circling. Neck circling exercises tend to grind down the cervical discs in addition to impinging on nerves and arteries. If you are doing neck rolls, do only a half circle—side, forward, side, forward, etc.

Questionable Shoulder Exercises

It has been estimated that 80 percent of college students have round shoulders; therefore, exercises which promote this condition should be avoided. Such things as push-ups, chinning, and forward-arm circling strengthen and shorten the already shortened pectoral (chest) muscles and should be avoided, *unless* they are balanced by activities which will stretch those muscles and strengthen the upper back and posterior shoulder muscles. Avoid doing arm circles with your palms down because the humerus impinges on the coracoacromial ligament and causes degenerative changes in the joint.

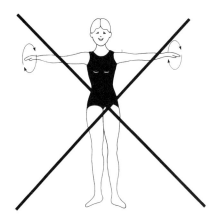

FIGURE 3.6 Arm circles with palms down

Questionable Foot and Leg Exercises

Deep Knee Bending. Doing these may damage the knee joint by pinching the synovial membrane, which provides lubrication of the joint, or by stretching the knee ligaments. Exercises which cause the knee to bend more than 90° such as the duck walk, Russian bear dance, and squat thrust are among those which should be avoided. Half knee bends (90° knee flexion) are acceptable, but the feet should always be directly under the knees to prevent a twist of the joint.

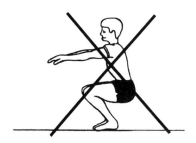

FIGURE 3.7 Deep knee bends

Splits. Doing or attempting to do the "splits" can cause serious damage. Most individuals are not anatomically built to assume this position, nor do they have a need to be so flexible in this area.

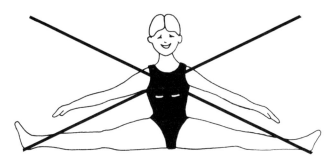

FIGURE 3.8 Splits

Standing on Tiptoe. Rising on the toes and maintaining this position strengthens and shortens the "calf" but stretches the plantar structures of the feet and weakens the arch. Part of the stretching can be eliminated by keeping the feet inverted (point toes in) when you stand on your tiptoes. Exercises which dorsiflex the foot (bring the toes toward the knee) should also be used to help maintain muscular balance and keep the calf from becoming too tight.

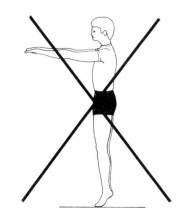

FIGURE 3.9 Standing on tiptoes

Questionable Flexibility Exercises

Standing Toe-Touch. This subject is a controversial one, but since it probably is better to err on the side of caution, it is mentioned here. Some people frown on the practice of stretching the hamstrings (posterior leg muscles) and lower back muscles by doing a standing toe-touch exercise. The usual method is to stand with straight legs, and try to touch the floor or toes by bouncing. It is felt that this exercise might lead to back strain and sciatica (because the sciatic nerve is stretched).

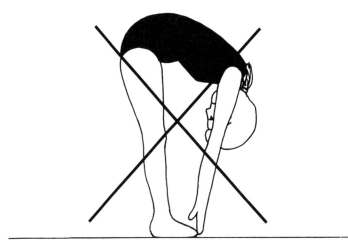

FIGURE 3.10 Standing toe-touch

The same exercise, done in a long-sitting position, would be less apt to damage structures because the body attains less momentum in the absence of gravity; therefore, the stretching force is less strenuous. Even this exercise can be hazardous. Back experts recommend stretching only one leg at a time; the other knee should be bent up toward the chest or out toward the side.

Frequently one hears or reads that toe touching is a good abdominal exercise. This is not true. It is a flexibility exercise and will not strengthen the abdominal muscles.

Hurdler's Stretch. Sitting in this unnatural position places stress on the knee joint and surrounding soft tissue. Also, it may cause a strain in the groin. Sitting with the foot placed toward the groin and the knee out is a much safer position. Use the "back-saver stretch" described under the "standing toe-touch."

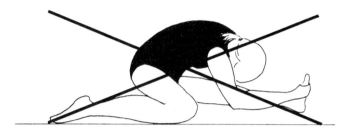

FIGURE 3.11 Hurdler's stretch

Knee Stretch. Sitting on your heels places stress on the knee joint and surrounding soft tissue.

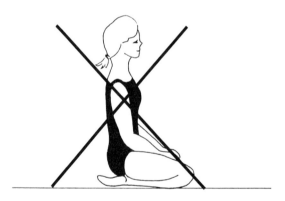

FIGURE 3.12 Knee stretch

Yoga Sitting. Assuming this unnatural position also places undue stress on the knee joint and surrounding soft tissue, and may cause a strain in the groin area.

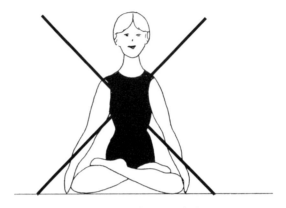

FIGURE 3.13 Yoga sitting

Plough. Resting the entire body weight on the neck and shoulders promotes head forward by stretching muscles and ligaments of the cervical and dorsal spine. If you wish to lower your head and elevate your feet, lie on a tilt board with your feet elevated.

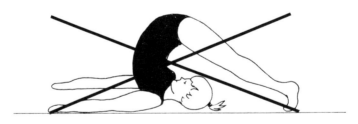

FIGURE 3.14 Plough

PRINCIPLES OF EXERCISE

When you begin an exercise program, do not expect to reach an adequate level of physical fitness immediately as it takes time and effort to bring about physiological changes. How much time and effort will depend upon your present status and your training program—the type of exercise as well as the frequency, intensity, and time (FIT principle). The program, directed toward the improvement of the five health-related fitness components, should be individually and systematically designed with you in mind. Whatever the program, you must follow the basic physiological principles of overload and adaptation, progression, and specificity.

Overload and Adaptation Principle

Your body systems tend to adapt to your daily routine—they become conditioned to meet these demands and no more. To improve this condition *make the systems (such as the heart, lungs, and muscles) "work" beyond the daily demand so that the amount of work being done is near maximum.* When your body has adapted to this new work level, increase the load until eventually your desired working level is reached. The overload (load beyond normal requirements) can be in the form of added weight or resistance, more repetitions, longer work periods, or a greater range of motion. It depends upon which of the five fitness components is being developed.

There is a *target zone* for (1) *frequency* (how often you exercise), (2) *intensity* (how much effort you put forth), and (3) *time* (how long you exercise), which is optimum for each individual for each component of fitness. If you exercise below the *threshold level* (the minimum amount of exercise necessary to build physical fitness), no change will occur. Likewise, exercising beyond the upper limits of the target zone will not bring good results because of injury and fatigue factors.

Progression Principle

Although the overload and adaptation principle is used to bring about changes in your body, you must gradually progress from what is considered to be a light work load for you to a heavy one. It is necessary to measure your current fitness status, since the beginning work load should be based upon this. Continue to measure your progress regularly in order to gradually increase your work load as the body adapts to each new change. A systematic program of gradually increasing the exercise difficulty (such as progressing from a bent knee push-up to an extended push-up or from a roll-down to a "crunch") will help prevent injuries, muscle soreness, and discouragement. You cannot become fit overnight. It will require four to six weeks of work before marked improvement is achieved.

Specificity Principle

When exercise is specific, it will develop only that fitness component it is designed to develop and only the body part that is being used. Weight training exercises are not designed to develop flexibility nor is jogging designed to develop arm strength. Select exercises to involve the specific areas you want to change. If you want to build strength, do heavy resistance work; if you want to improve your cardiovascular endurance, involve large muscle groups to bring about an increased heart rate for extended periods of time, if you want to develop flexibility in your lower back, perform exercises that stretch these muscles. Exercises are also "task specific." You should train the muscles with the same speed and coordination that they will need in the task. For example, select workouts that will train you for a specific event. If you want to swim distances, for part of your workout train by swimming; if you want to run distances, running should be a part of your training regimen.

TYPES OF MUSCULAR CONTRACTIONS

Muscles contract in these ways: they may shorten, with the ends being brought toward the center (*concentric*); they may lengthen, with the ends moving away from the center (*eccentric*); or they may hold, without changing length. For example, when doing a push-up exercise the movement upward uses a concentric contraction of the elbow extensors; the movement downward uses an eccentric contraction. Contractions involving changes in muscle length (concentric and eccentric) are referred to as *isotonic* or dynamic contractions. Those involving no change in muscle length (a held contraction) are referred to as *isometric* or static contractions. For example, in the push-up exercise if you pause on the upward movement and hold the body in the mid position for a few seconds, the triceps muscles will be contracting isometrically. All types of contractions can develop strength and muscular endurance, but only the isotonic type can improve cardiovascular endurance and flexibility.

TRAINING EFFECT

You can achieve a desirable level of physical fitness by selecting exercises with your particular goals in mind, setting up a training program, following the general suggestions for exercising, and using the basic physiological principles of training. After you have reached your goals, you should continue a physical-maintenance program if you want to remain at your achieved level of fitness.

Muscular Strength

Any of the three basic types of muscle training programs—isotonic, isometric, or isokinetic—can be used to develop muscular strength. Regardless of the program used, the principles of exercise—overload and adaptation, progression, and specificity—apply.

Isotonic exercises are those that require the muscle to shorten and/or lengthen and the joint (or extremity) to move. Weightlifting is the most common exercise that is used to build strength; however, it has little effect on the cardiovascular system. Lifting 70 percent of the maximum weight you can lift in one effort in three sets of five to eight repetitions three or four days a week (every other day) will develop strength. **Isometric** exercises are those that contract muscles but do not move joints or extremities. If you hold a maximum contraction against an immovable object for five seconds five to seven times a session (allow two minutes for recovery between efforts) three or four days a week (every other day), you would become stronger. Training sessions can be held daily if you do not develop muscular soreness. An **isokinetic** exercise involves moving resistance through a range of motion on a device or machine which matches the resistance to the force applied by your muscles and controls the speed of movement. The Cybex and Exergenie are examples of this type of machine. Machines such as the Nautilus and Universal (some stations) provide variable resistance but do not control the speed. See chapters 4 and 5 for information concerning exercises and training programs.

Muscular Endurance

This second component of fitness is helped somewhat by muscular strength because if you are strong, you may be able to continue the exercise for extended periods of time. However, strength and endurance are not the same so training programs are different. This component of fitness may be developed through isotonic or isometric exercises. To improve isotonic muscular endurance, you should work against light to moderate resistance, doing a large number of repetitions (15 to 25). Progressively overloading the muscles either in weight or repetitions can be done by weight training or by doing selected calisthenics—for example, push-ups for arm muscular endurance and jumping rope or doing jumping jacks for leg muscular endurance. To improve isometric muscular endurance, contract isometrically and hold the contraction for increasing periods of time, up to 20 percent longer than your anticipated need in the activity for which you are specifically training.

Cardiovascular Endurance

This fitness component is developed by performing activities which apply stress to the heart as well as to the circulatory and respiratory systems. It should be maintained continuously and rhythmically, and may be either *aerobic* (with oxygen), *anaerobic* (without oxygen), or a combination of the two.

The aerobic activity must be performed frequently (at least three times per week), with intensity (heart rate should be at least 60 percent of the working capacity), and for appropriate periods of time (from 15 minutes to 60 minutes, depending on intensity). Examples of suitable aerobic activities are swimming, cycling, cross country skiing, and jogging.

To develop cardiovascular fitness using anaerobic training you must also follow the FIT principle. You must workout at least three days a week and raise your heart rate to at least 70 percent of its working capacity. The workout should last at least 15 minutes and be divided into alternate periods of "work" and "rest" (*interval training*)—keep the heart rate up for 20 to 30 seconds (work) and then do slow exercise for 60 to 90 seconds (rest for three times as long as you worked) and continue to repeat. Examples of appropriate activities are sports such as racquetball, team handball, and badminton, and sprints in running, swimming, and cycling.

Your initial level of fitness will determine your beginning workload, but the interrelation among frequency, intensity, and time makes it possible to be flexible in setting up your program. The consensus of opinion of many researchers is that 15 minutes is the *minimum* amount of time for you to keep your heart rate elevated to build cardiovascular endurance. The general rule is that low intensity workouts must be of longer duration than high intensity ones; however, if you are a completely sedentary individual, elevating your heart rate above the resting level for 10 minutes may be of some benefit. Most experts recommend 60 percent work for 45–60 minutes, 70 percent work for 30–45 minutes, 80 percent work for 15–20 minutes. Short exercise periods with the higher working heart rate are for the young (under 30) and healthy adults or the well trained athletes; long work periods with lower working heart rate are for those with low levels of fitness or who are older. Know your fitness level and plan a regimen (aerobic, anaerobic, or a combination) that will allow you to improve your cardiovascular endurance, avoid injury and muscle soreness, and maintain your interest.

Flexibility

The fourth fitness component, flexibility, is developed and maintained by regularly moving body parts through a full range of motion, thus stretching the muscles and the tendons that surround the joint(s). Because of their elasticity and extensibility, muscles and tendons can be lengthened temporarily or on a more permanent basis. The objective, of course, is to achieve the more permanent type of lengthening.

Flexibility exercises can be done alone or with a partner. They may be done *ballistically* (producing momentum by bobbing or bouncing) or *statically* (contracting muscles and holding the position), and they may be *passive* (having a partner or outside force move the body segment) or *active* (contracting the muscles opposing the ones you are trying to stretch). Even though all of these may be effective, ballistic and passive stretching are more hazardous because they may overstretch the connective tissues and can cause injury. If passive stretch is used (unless it is administered by a qualified therapist), it should be combined with active static in what is called an *active-assistive* stretch. For best results:

1. Perform the exercise daily. Stretching is a necessary part of the warm-up and cool-down phases of the workouts.
2. Apply the three principles of exercise—overload and adaptation, progression, and specificity.

3. Perform the exercise slowly. Do not overstretch by forcing the movement to the point of pain.
4. Hold the static stretch in the lengthened position for 15 to 30 seconds.
5. Relax the muscle that is to be stretched immediately before the stretch to make the exercise more effective.
6. Keep forceful types of movements to a minimum. If you use a ballistic stretch, precede it with active static stretching, reach gently, and use it on healthy joints only.

Body Composition

Body composition, the fifth fitness component, refers to the individual elements that make up total body mass. The element that will probably be a primary concern to you is fat. Women possess more fat relative to body weight than men; however, their bodies react to physical activity and diet (the means to alter body composition) in the same ways. Experts believe that you cannot change the number of fat cells, unless you have them surgically removed, but you can change their size.

With regular exercise and proper diet, the lean body weight will increase while the fat body weight decreases. The rate and amount of change is largely dependent on the type of training program, with gains in lean weight being facilitated by strength training and losses in fat weight being facilitated by endurance training. A well planned exercise program will combine aerobic activity such as jogging, dancing, and cycling with localized exercises such as calisthenics and/or weight training.

It may also be necessary to combine the exercise program with a calorie restricted diet to achieve the desired results. See chapter 6 for information concerning the diet.

CALCULATING TARGET HEART RATE

One method of calculating the intensity needed to put your workout in the target zone is described here. (A worksheet is found in the Appendix, Chart III.) First determine your resting heart rate (RHR). The best time to check this is in the morning before you get out of bed. Apply light pressure with the tips of the first two fingers on the inside of the wrist just below the base of the thumb (radial artery) or on the side of the neck on either side of your "Adam's Apple" on the carotid artery. Count the pulse for 60 seconds (begin counting with 0); count three separate times to get a more accurate reading. Then establish your maximum heart rate (MHR) by subtracting your age from 220 (the estimated maximum heart rate−EMHR). For example 20-year old Sammy has a maximum heart rate of 200 (220−20). If her resting heart rate

(RHR) is 72, she can find her working heart rate (WHR) by subtracting the RHR from the MHR. If she chooses to work at the lower limit of her working capacity (for example 60 percent) she will multiply the WHR by .60 and then add her RHR to the total (see sample calculation).

$$
\begin{array}{rl}
220 & \text{(EMHR)} \\
-20 & \text{(age)} \\
\hline
200 & \text{(MHR)} \\
-72 & \text{(RHR)} \\
\hline
128 & \text{(WHR)} \\
\times \quad .60 & \text{(lower limit of working capacity)} \\
\hline
76.80 & \\
+72.00 & \text{(RHR)} \\
\hline
148.8 & \text{or 149 beats per minute (lower limit of target zone)}
\end{array}
$$

Exercises for Fitness, Figure, and Physique

4

PRETEST

1. What activities can be used to develop cardiovascular fitness?
2. How do you design a training program to improve cardiovascular fitness?
3. How do you design a training program to improve your muscle endurance and strength?
4. What exercises can be used to develop specific components of health related fitness?
5. What can you do to improve your figure/physique?

In the decade of the 1970s, millions of Americans appeared to discover physical activity. They walked, swam, cycled, jogged, danced, played games, and did calisthenics. At the end of the 70s, one-half of the Americans aged 20 or older reported that they exercised on a regular basis.[1] In the 80s, 54 percent of the adults interviewed in a study done for *American Health* reported that they exercised regularly.[2] They are interested in exercise because they believe that by participating in physical activity their lives will be transformed.

Many individuals choose to participate in exercise activities, rather than sports activities, because being an "athlete" is not a prerequisite, the dollar cost can be minimal, and one can work alone or with others. Also, exercises can be more easily adjusted to the environment (primarily time and space factors) and be designed to meet specific needs and interests. Exercises can be combined in a variety of ways to form a good training program. You may elect to design your own or use some of the examples given in chapter 5.

CARDIOVASCULAR FITNESS

Aerobic Exercises

Aerobic means "with oxygen." Aerobic exercises are those that require large quantities of oxygen for extended periods. They characteristically involve covering long distances slowly as compared to covering short distances rapidly (anaerobic). Recommendations concerning aerobic training programs are as follows:

1. Frequency—Work out a minimum of three days a week.
2. Intensity—Elevate your heart rate to at least 60 percent of your maximum heart rate reserve.
3. Duration—Keep your heart rate elevated for at least 15 continuous minutes. The duration depends upon the intensity of the activity; the lower intensity should be conducted for a longer period of time, perhaps as long as 60 minutes. Low to moderate intensity of longer duration is recommended for the average adult who is not in training for an athletic event.
4. Activity—Choose an activity that uses large muscle groups, that can be maintained continuously, and are rhythmical and aerobic in nature. Examples of suitable activities are: running/jogging, walking/hiking, swimming, skating, cycling, cross-country skiing, and various endurance game activities.[3]

Generally, for the average college student, a 60 percent level of intensity is considered to be the lower end of the continuum, and this level should be maintained for 30 to 40 minutes. If work at a moderate level (70 percent) is preferred, it should be continued at this rate for 20 to 30 minutes. Working at a high level (80 percent) requires 15 to 20 continuous minutes.

You can plan a more effective program if you know your present level of aerobic fitness. One test that you can use is the *12-minute run*. The objective is to see how much distance you can cover in 12 minutes of running, jogging, and/or walking. According to Cooper, a college age female running 1.19 miles in this time frame has a "fair" level of aerobic fitness. Covering 1.3 miles gives a "good" rating, 1.44 miles is in the "excellent" category, and 1.52 miles ranks as "superior." For males in this age range, 1.38 miles is in the "fair" category, 1.57 miles rates as "good," 1.73 miles denotes "excellent," and 1.87 miles gives a "superior" rating.[4] Another test that you can take is the *1½ mile run* which is discussed in chapter 1.

Pulse Rated Programs. Cardiovascular endurance training can be monitored by measuring oxygen uptake or by measuring heart rate. The former requires laboratory equipment so, for most people, checking their heart rate is more practical. For example, if you are a moderately active 20 year old with a resting heart rate of 70, 70 percent of your working heart rate will be 161 beats per minute (bpm). If you choose to work at 80 percent, your working heart rate will be 174 bpm. (See formula on page 44.) Select an activity that will keep your heart rate between 160 and 170 bpm for approximately 20 minutes. If you are a sedentary individual with a resting heart rate of 80, work at a lower level at the beginning; 150 to 160 (about 60 percent) bpm may be of suitable itensity initially. To check to see if you are going too fast too soon, talk during the exercise. If you cannot do this comfortably, you are working at a level that is too high. If you can carry on a normal conversation, keep working. Monitor your heart rate after five minutes and again after 10 minutes. If it is above your target heart rate range (THR), slow down; if it is below the THR, increase the intensity. With practice you will learn to pace yourself so that you can stay within the range. Immediately upon stopping, count your pulse (begin with 0) for 10 seconds and multiply by six. This is your actual exercise pulse.

Running programs are frequently used to develop cardiovascular fitness. As with any exercise program you should warm-up and cool-down slowly; include stretching exercises for the arms, legs, and back. Two currently popular ones are:

1. *Continuous Slow Running* (*Jogging*) which involves running a long distance at a relatively slow pace is a versatile exercise. You can do it alone or in groups, inside or outside, on a track or down the road, and at any time of day. Not only does it develop the cardiovascular and respiratory systems but exercises the arms as well as the legs, and has a firming effect on muscle groups throughout the body. It is a quick way to get the training effect started. You set the rate at a slow, steady pace, and a distance or length of time that seems appropriate for you.

2. *Rebound-Running.* Jog-bounce (termed rebound-run) on a mini-trampoline is another form of aerobic exercise. These rebounders absorb the impact of landing and do not place as much stress on your joints; jogging on a mini-tramp is not as intense as jogging on a track but it is at least equal to walking.[5] For the relatively unfit it may be a good way to start a fitness program but it is difficult for fit individuals to get their heart rates up to the target zones on a trampoline. As your fitness level improves, the rebounder may not work you hard enough to improve your aerobic capacity unless light handweights are held to increase the workload.

Walking, an easy exercise to start and continue, is a low intensity method of training. It is for those who cannot run, choose to not run, or need to work into a conditioning program gradually. The benefits are basically the same as those for running, but it takes longer to achieve a training effect as the heart rate does not rise as high as it does for the more vigorous activities. If you maintain your heart rate at 60 percent working capacity for at least 15 minutes, you would see results sooner but that is difficult to do in a walking program unless you have lead a rather sedentary life-style. Walking faster, swinging your arms vigorously, walking up hills, or carrying light handweights will increase your workload. Older adults can get a training effect with as little as 40 percent working capacity but it needs to be maintained for 45 to 60 minutes.

Aerobic dance exercise was pioneered in the early 1970s and quickly became a popular activity, primarily with women. In the 80s, many men discovered that it was a fun way to exercise and became interested in this type of cardiovascular workout. This activity utilizes a series of specially choreographed routines which are combinations of various dance steps and locomotor and non-locomotor movements. As with all workouts you should warm-up and stretch before and after the exercise.

There are several levels and types of workouts, ranging from "nonimpact" aerobics (these are questionable as movement is limited) to "Rambo" aerobics. The latter requires you to be in top physical condition and desirous of a serious exhausting workout. Somewhere between these two programs lies "low-impact" aerobics that became popular in the mid 1980s because many participants were being injured in regular aerobic dance and exercise programs. Common injuries were shin splints, stress fractures, and tendinitis. In the low impact workout one foot remains in contact with the floor during the aerobic portion and large upper body movements are combined with low kicks, high steps, side-to-side movements, and lunges. A high impact workout may be more intense but a well designed low impact one can get your pulse rate into the target zone. Holding light handweights (begin with one-half pound) during a workout can raise the level of intensity.

Dancing can be an effective means of achieving cardiovascular fitness. Some preliminary studies by researchers have shown that carefully designed folk and social dance routines can be used to improve your level of cardiovascular fitness.[6] Dance routines, such as "Social Dance Aerobics," which allow you to achieve the intensity and duration needed for a training effect are available on video.

Aquacize, working out in the water, can be a nice change of pace. This may be preferable to exercising on land, particularly if you have a weight bearing problem, because of the buoying effect of the water. The water offers resistance to the movement and can cause the heart rate to reach an even higher level than when you do the same exercise on land.

The routine would be much like those of any other workout—begin with a warm-up, follow with muscular conditioning, have your aerobic workout, and end with a cool-down. Get the body part(s) you want to exercise under water so that there will be more resistance—stand in waist- to chest-deep water to run, dance, twist, and do calisthenics. Grasp the side of the pool to do other exercises. Increase resistance by using devices such as fins, paddles, mitten boards, or empty plastic jugs. Working out in the water (do not use the hot tub) is a good general training routine, but bone density will not be improved as much as in weight bearing exercises.

Jumping rope can be a very demanding exercise because the leg muscles (large muscles demand more oxygen than small ones) do the bulk of the work. If you do not have the skill to jump rope, this routine might not be effective for you because you cannot keep your heart rate in the target heart rate range for an extended period of time. However, skill can be developed as can a rope jump routine that can be an effective program for achieving a training effect. A workout can be fitted rather easily into a demanding schedule as you need only a rope, proper shoes, space, and a brief period of time (10 to 20 minutes). This can be a very strenuous workout, so begin working at a low level.

Cooper's Aerobic Point System was introduced in the 1960s and refined in the 1970s.[7] Aerobic exercises were quantified by means of a point system and goals set for men (30 points per week for those under 30 years of age) and women (24 points per week for those under 30 years of age). The type of aerobic activity (28 different activities were quantified) one chooses to use does not matter but reaching the goal is important. If you get the established number of points each week, your fitness is good. Top ranked aerobic activities, listed in order, are cross-country skiing, swimming, jogging or running (covering a mile in less than nine minutes), outdoor cycling, indoor cycling, walking, and aerobic dance.[8]

Anaerobic Exercises

Anaerobics means "without oxygen." Anaerobic capacity is defined as the ability to continue to maintain strenuous muscular contractions without using the oxygen that you are breathing. There is a fine line between anaerobic and aerobic exercises. The determining factor is your fitness level in relation to the physical requirement of the activity; however, if you run the 100 yard dash, sprint up a flight of stairs, make a concerted effort to break a wrestling hold, or beat out a slow roller in a softball game, you will probably be relying upon your anaerobic capacity. A training program utilizing anaerobic activities can be used very effectively to improve your cardiovascular endurance. See chapter 5 for additional information.

Training. Training anaerobically requires the use of interval training, intense work periods interspersed with rest periods to help the body adapt to stressful demands. Work periods of 90 to 100 percent intensity should range from 20 seconds to two minutes (depending upon the activity demands). The longer the work period, the longer the rest period. For example, a 20 second workout requires at least a 40 second rest period; a 60 second workout could require a four-minute rest period. Too, the longer the work period, the fewer the number of periods per session. Five interval training periods of one minute performed three to four times a week should result in an improvement in the cardiovascular system.

Active sports such as badminton, team handball, and basketball are usually anaerobic. Cycling can be an anaerobic activity if you alternate pedaling fast and pedaling slowly. Activities that require you to go "all out" for a short period of time are generally anaerobic. If you are trying to improve your level of cardiovascular endurance, keep the rest periods balanced with your work periods—do not take a long break!

Interval Running is a type of training that consists of alternating a work period with a rest period. Three variables are involved: the distance to be run, the time needed to run the distance, and the rest period (either a specified time or distance) between each run. You may alter any of these to arrange your workout so that it consists of alternating sprinting with jogging or walking. You may choose to run 5 repetitions of 50 yards at full speed with a 25-yard jog between each repetition, or run 4 repetitions of 100 yards at full speed with a 20-second walk interval between each of the repetitions. Longer distances can be covered. You may decide to run two repetitions of one mile each in eight minutes, with a three-minute walk rest interval between the repetitions.

Acceleration Running involves moving from jogging to striding, to sprinting, to walking. The distance may vary as you move from the slow pace (jog 30 yards), to a faster pace (stride 30 yards), to moving at full speed for 30 yards. Follow this with 40 or 50 yards of walking before beginning the routine again. Repeat several times.

Interval Aerobics is not a new type of training but interval aerobics is a relatively new concept in the United States. Limited research findings show that a well designed aerobic interval training program can produce cardiovascular training effects and reduce body fat.[9] Also, this type of training was found to be less boring and less fatiguing than continuous exercise. A routine always begins with a five- to ten-minute warm-up and ends with a cool-down. Intense intervals of work (seven to ten of three to five minutes duration) are interspersed with rest intervals (walking) of two to three minutes duration.

STRENGTH AND MUSCULAR ENDURANCE

Who needs muscular fitness? You do if you want to be a totally fit individual. Anyone can develop strength and muscular endurance but not necessarily to the same levels. Men and women can improve their muscular systems by following the same principles of training; however, the degree of muscle hypertrophy in women is much less than that in men because, in general, women have less muscle mass and lower levels of testosterone.

Progressive Resistance Exercises

Throughout a weight training program the work load must be increased gradually, progressing from a relatively light resistance to a heavy one, in order to ensure continued improvement in muscular strength or endurance. These progressive resistance exercises (P.R.E.), which may be isotonic or isokinetic, allow you to develop muscular endurance or strength by precisely regulating the degree of muscular stress for the muscle group desired. Progress is easy to follow as more weight is added and/or the number of repetitions increases, and P.R.E. tends to be less boring than isometric exercises. P.R.E. involves the use of resistance such as free weights, springs, elastic tubes, wall pulleys, and devices or machines like ergometers. They also involve the use of variable resistance machines, such as the Nautilus and Universal, and isokinetic machines.

Terms. You should become well acquainted with some of the common terms used in resistance exercises. *Repetitions* (*reps*) refer to the number of times a movement is repeated. A *set* means a group of successive reps without an intervening rest. *Resistance* refers to the amount of weight being moved, or the resistance overcome. *Repetition maximum* (*RM*) is the maximum weight which can be lifted a specified number of times using maximum (100%) muscular exertion; for example, eight RM means that the set consisted of eight reps at maximum exertion. Eight-3/4 RM means that the set consisted of eight reps at 75 percent of your maximum exertion.

Weight Training Exercises

There is no single program that is best for all, so do not attempt to duplicate one that is designed for someone else. Before beginning, ask yourself, "What muscles do I want to develop and for what purpose?" The basic design of your program should be determined by your answer. When designing a program to improve your figure or physique it is important to include exercises for all major muscle groups so that a pleasing body symmetry is achieved. If you wish to add pounds to your frame, not only is it important to select the right exercises but proper diet is also essential. (See chapter 6.)

Safety. Safety (particularly when using free-weights) must be a primary concern if you want to avoid injuries and sore muscles. Factors to consider are the warm-up period (discussed on page 2), weight selection, proper execution of the exercise, intensity of the workout, and frequency of workouts.

Selecting the correct weight depends upon a variety of factors including your age, weight, strength, and overall condition as well as the exercise itself. Each muscle group has a different strength capacity—leg muscles tend to be stronger than those in your arms so you can handle more weight with your legs. Some exercises, such as pull-overs, afford poor leverage so only light weights should be used. Use a modified trial and error method to select your beginning weight. Predetermine that you will do three sets of six or eight reps of a particular exercise. If you do this easily, the weight is too light for you; if it is difficult, the weight is too heavy. For some of you who are lifting free weights, the bar alone may be a good beginning weight. You should not add weight until you can perform the exercise correctly, and then it should be added in small increments. Do not go too fast too soon.

Proper execution is a must if you are to avoid injuries. It is vitally important that each exercise be performed throughout the specific muscle group's full range of muscular activity and that each repetition be executed correctly. Each repetition should start from the *prestretched position* (with the muscle elongated) and be executed concentrically (shorten the muscles) for about two seconds and then eccentrically (lengthen the muscles) for about four seconds. Large muscle groups (back, chest, hips, legs) are generally exercised before the smaller muscle groups (neck, elbow, wrist, ankle). When using free weights use spotters, especially on bench presses. When doing a dead lift or picking up a free weight use the "4" rather than the "7" position when lifting—this means flex your knees and hips but keep your back straight ("4") rather than keeping legs straight and bending the back ("7"). Maintain good body alignment: keep your pelvis stabilized. All movements must be executed smoothly; there should be no jerking or heaving. It is customary to exhale during the exertion of the movement and to inhale as the weight is lowered. Do *not* hold your breath.

The *level of intensity* must be carefully monitored, especially at the beginning of a program. If you are interested in developing *strength,* a relatively safe practice is to begin with a light weight and perform three sets of eight reps. Later, progress to nine reps but keep the same weight. When this becomes easy, move to 10 reps and then to 12. At that point, increase the weight and decrease the reps to eight. Work up to 12 reps again, increase the weight, and decrease to eight reps. The rate of progression should be faster if you are working with your leg muscles as opposed to your arm muscles. Rest a minimum of two minutes (more will be necessary for high intensity workouts) between sets. Another frequently utilized system is the De Lorme P.R.E. program in which the amount of weight increases from one set to the next. You determine your reps (eight for example) and begin by lifting 50 percent of your RM. You progress to eight reps of 75 percent RM, and end with eight reps at RM. Others involved in a P.R.E. program use the Oxford System in which the amount of weight being lifted decreases from set to set. You begin with RM, then use 75 percent RM, and finish at 50 percent RM.

Muscular endurance is improved by performing a high number of reps (15 to 25) with light to moderate resistance (30 to 50 percent RM). You may select a weight by trial and error. If you follow this procedure, realistically appraise your fitness level and then select a light weight—perhaps about one-third of your body weight if you are lifting with your legs. Perform three sets of 20 reps with this weight; rest for about two minutes between sets. When you feel that this is not a sufficient workload, increase the amount of weight or do 25 reps with the same weight.

Frequency of Workouts. How often should you lift? The consensus of opinion is that you should work out every other day (allow a 48-hour rest period). Some athletes may work out every day but they usually work on different muscle groups each day; perhaps the legs one day and the upper body the next. Your muscles need time to recover.

Weight Training Workouts. To make significant gains in muscular development, the specific exercises should be performed in three sets every other day. The length of the workout may vary (from 30 minutes to two hours) depending upon the type and number of exercises being done. If you are working on all major muscle groups in one workout, alternate among lower-limb, trunk, and upper-limb exercises. Two workouts a week will maintain your level of fitness once you have reached it.

Exercises With Free Weights

You can find specific exercises for strength or muscular endurance in weight training books and charts that usually accompany a weight machine. The exercises in this chapter are only a few of the many used to develop muscular endurance and strength. Dumbbells, pulleys, or other resistance exercises can be substituted in many of these exercises.

1. *Two-arm* (*Biceps*) Curl—used to develop the flexors of the elbow. Stand erect, arms at sides

Place feet shoulder width apart

Point toes straight ahead

Face palms forward

Place hands shoulder width apart

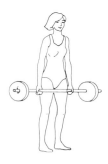

a. Begin

Curl bar slowly and steadily to shoulder

Exhale while raising weight

Keep elbows close to but not touching body

Return slowly and steadily to starting position

Inhale while lowering weight

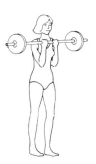

b. Execute

2. *Upright Rowing*—used to develop the flexors of the elbow and the muscles of the shoulders and upper back.
Stand erect

Place feet shoulder width apart

Point toes straight ahead

Face palms toward body

Keep hands close together

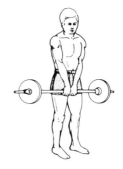

a. Begin

Lift bar slowly and steadily to chin

Exhale while raising weight

Keep bar close to body

Keep elbows higher than hands

Return slowly and steadily to starting position

Inhale while lowering weight

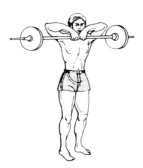

b. Execute

3. *Bench Press*—used to develop extensors of the elbows and flexors of the shoulders and the chest.
Have a spotter

Lie supine on a bench

Place feet on bench shoulder width apart (keep arch out of the back)

Turn palms away from face

Place hands about shoulder width apart; place thumbs under bar

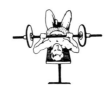

a. Begin

Push the bar slowly and steadily until arms are extended

Exhale on the extension

Return slowly and steadily to starting position

Inhale while lowering weight

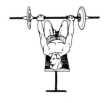

b. Execute

4. *Shoulder Press*—is used to develop the arm extensors. Stand erect

Place feet shoulder width apart

Point toes straight ahead

Start weight at chest height

Face palms away from body

Place hands shoulder width apart

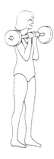

a. Begin

Push the bar slowly and steadily until arms are fully extended

Exhale while raising weight

Keep weight in line with center of gravity

Do not arch back

Return slowly and steadily to starting position

Inhale while lowering weight

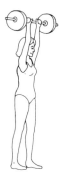

b. Execute

5. *Half Knee Squats*—used to develop the muscles of the upper parts of the thighs.

Stand erect

Spread feet shoulder width apart

Point toes straight ahead

Face palms forward

Place hands farther than shoulder width apart

Rest bar on shoulders

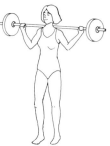

a. Begin

Squat slowly and steadily

Bend knees to 90° angle

Inhale while body is being lowered

Pause briefly; take several deep breaths

Return slowly and steadily to starting position

Exhale while raising body

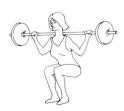

b. Execute

6. *Heel-Raises*—used to develop the calf muscles in the lower leg. Stand erect

Place feet shoulder width apart

Point toes in slightly

Face palms forward

Place hands farther apart than shoulder width apart

Rest bar on shoulders

(Place balls of feet on two inch high board for greater range of motion.)

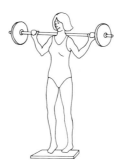

a. Begin

Rise on tiptoes slowly and steadily

Exhale while raising weight

Extend legs fully; toes turned in slightly

Keep weight over base of support; do not lean

Hold for one second

Return slowly and steadily until heels touch floor.

Inhale as weight is lowered

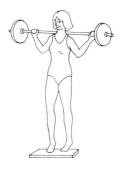

b. Execute

Exercises with Dumbbells

Most exercises that can be performed with a barbell can be duplicated with a dumbbell. The following are two examples. (Tins of food—such as 20 ounces of peaches, sand filled plastic bottles, or books may be substituted for regular dumbbells.)

7. *Side Bends*—used to develop lateral flexors.
   Stand erect; comfortable side stride position

   Hold dumbbell at side

   Face palms toward body

   Place free hand on hip

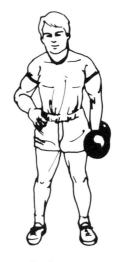

a. Begin

Bend slowly and steadily to the side

Do not lean forward or backward

Return to starting position

Repeat using other arm and bend in opposite direction

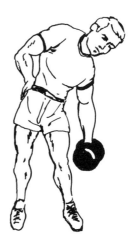

b. Execute

8. *Flying Motions*—used to develop shoulders, upper chest, and back. Lie supine on flat bench

Place feet on bench shoulder width apart (keep arch out of the back)

Hold dumbbells with palms facing up

Extend arms in line with shoulders

Partially flex the elbows

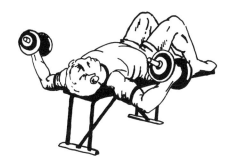

a. Begin

Cross arms slowly and steadily over the chest

Alternate arms in crossing so that one is uppermost one time and the other the next

Exhale while lifting weight

Return to starting position

Inhale while lowering weight

(Some individuals prefer to alternate arms—one arm goes up as the other comes down.)

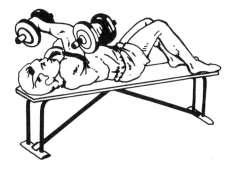

b. Execute

CALISTHENICS

The term calisthenics generally refers to the more traditional exercises, such as sit-ups and push-ups, which can be done with little or no equipment. They may be isotonic (suitable for developing isotonic muscular endurance, isotonic strength, and flexibility) or isometric (suitable for developing isometric strength and isometric muscular endurance). You can develop strength with isotonic exercises only if your body parts or body weight provides an overload for you. Some exercises such as jumping jacks and leg changes may be used to improve your aerobic capacity. As with any workout, the results depend upon your fitness level, the exercise, and the frequency, intensity, and time devoted to the workout.

Calisthenic exercises probably number in the thousands, but only a few have been selected for inclusion in this book. Your instructor may suggest additional ones, and you may wish to seek still others to vary your program. From those selected to meet your personal needs, you may find that combining them into a fixed daily routine has several advantages. With intelligent selection, the fixed routine allows the important body parts to be exercised regularly. Such a routine saves time by eliminating the "what-shall-I-do today?" decision. Examples of two scientifically conceived routines, the *Royal Canadian Air Force Exercise Plans for Physical Fitness* and the *Continuous Exercise Routine,* are included in chapter 5.

SELECTED EXERCISES FOR PHYSICAL FITNESS

The repetitions noted for each exercise are suggested beginning levels. Start at this level and gradually increase the repetitions.

Strength and Endurance: Arms and Shoulders

9. *Wall Push-ups*—Stand facing a wall that is arm's length away. Extend your arms, place the palms of your hand flat on the walls at chest height. Keep your body in a straight line from head to feet as you slowly flex your arms and lean toward the wall until your face almost touches it. Slowly extend your arms. Keep your feet flat on the floor throughout the movement to stretch your calf muscles. Repeat eight to ten times.

10. *Negative Push-ups*—Assume a modified push-up position (see page 4) with your arms extended. Keep your body straight from head to knees as you slowly (take as much time as you can) lower yourself to the floor. Return to the up position in any way you choose. Repeat five times.

11. *Push-ups*—Assume the push-up position. Lower your body until your chest touches the floor, and return to the starting position, keeping your body straight. Repeat five times. (See page 5.)

12. *Pull-ups*—Hang (palms forward and shoulder width apart) from a low bar (may be placed across two chairs), heels on floor, with the body suspended at about a 45 degree angle. Pull up, keeping the body rigid, and touch your chest to the bar. Lower to the starting position. Repeat three times. (See page 3.)

13. *Isometric Hand-pull*—Tailor sit or stand. Keeping the arms at shoulder level, place hands under chin, with fingers extended. Turn one hand palm up and lock fingertips. Keeping the fingertips locked, try to pull the elbows apart. Hold for six seconds, relax, and repeat three times per day.

14. *Negative Pull-ups*—Stand on a stool that will allow you to grasp a high bar with your chin just over the bar. Step off the stool and hang, then extend your arms as slowly as you can until your arms are fully extended. Repeat three to five times.

Strength and Endurance: Abdominals

15. *Roll-downs*—(For persons who can not do sit-ups) Sit with the knees bent and the feet together. Fold your arms across your chest and roll down slowly, keeping the chin tucked to the chest. Relax on the floor, and then sit up any way you choose. Repeat ten times. (If you cannot do No. 16, do this one.)

16. *Crunches*—Repeat eight times. (See page 4.)

17. *Reverse Sit-ups*—Lie on your back, bend the knees, place the feet flat on the floor with arms at sides. Lift the knees to the chest, raising the hips off the floor. Return to the starting position. You may raise the knees toward the right shoulder and then to the left shoulder. Repeat four times.

18. *Pelvic Tilt*—Assume a supine position, with the knees bent and slightly apart. "Press" the spine down on the floor and hold for six seconds—tighten the abdominals and gluteals. Repeat three times, three times per day.

19. *Abdominal and Gluteal Set* (also for legs)—Stand tall, with the feet together, arms hanging loosely at the sides. Tighten the abdominals, gluteals, and thigh muscles. Keep the legs straight (not hyperextended), and tip the pelvis backward.

20. *Leg-up*—Lie supine and extend your right leg. Place your arms in an extended position at your sides. Bend your left hip at a 45° angle; keep your left foot on the floor. Lift the extended right leg off the floor six to 12 inches as you reach forward with your hands and roll your head and upper torso up from the floor. Keep the small of your back on the floor. Hold for ten seconds and then return to the supine position. Repeat three times with each leg.

21. *Hanging Leg Raises*—Grasp a high bar with palms facing forward, shoulder width apart. Hang from the bar as you slowly flex your hips and knees. Raise the knees as high as you can toward your chest. Hold for six seconds, lower slowly, and repeat three times.

Strength and Endurance: Legs

22. *Stationary Leg Change*—Crouch on the floor, with your weight on your hands, left leg bent under the chest, right leg extended behind you. Alternate legs—bring right leg up while left leg goes back. Repeat, alternating right and left, 16 times.

23. *Stride Squat*—Stand tall, feet together. Take a long step forward with the left foot, touching the right knee to the floor. Return to the starting position, and step out with the other foot. Repeat, alternating left and right, eight times.

24. *Flat-foot Rock*—Stand in a wide side-stride position, with the toes pointing outward and the hands on the hips. Lower into a "squat" (knees flexed 90°) over one foot while keeping the other leg straight. Keep the feet in the same spot, and transfer the body from a "squat" over one foot to a "squat" over the other. Do not raise the body while changing position. Repeat, alternating right and left, four times.

25. *Isometric Leg Extensor*—Stand on a jump rope in a side-stride position with back erect, knees slightly flexed, and hands grasping rope at about knee level. Keep the back erect and arms straight while making an attempt to straighten your knees by pulling directly upward on the rope. Hold for six seconds, relax, and repeat three times, three times per day.

26. *Modified Knee Bends*—Stand in a side-stride position with feet about six inches apart. Kneel on the right knee while maintaining good posture. Return to starting position by extending left leg. Kneel on the right knee five times in succession. Repeat with left knee. Do not flex the supporting knee more than 90°. (You can maintain balance by holding on to something if you lack sufficient strength.)

Flexibility: Chest, Shoulders, Upper Back

(See pages 122, 123, and 133.)

27. *Arm Back*—Tailor sit or stand. Bend the elbows, keeping the arms at shoulder level and the palms down, under the chin. Push the elbows back, trying to bring the shoulder blades together, then return to starting position. Extend the arms, keeping them at shoulder level, and stretch them behind you. Return to original position. Repeat set four times. Keep your chin tucked and your head back.

28. *Prone Elbow Lift*—Lie in a prone position. Place the hands in the small of the back, palms upward. Raise the elbows and shoulders without moving the trunk and head; hold for four counts. Relax and repeat four times.

29. *Overhead Reach*—Sit in a chair, tailor sit on the floor, or stand erect. Extend your arms forward at shoulder height, keep your palms facing the ceiling. Keep the palms in this position as you slowly raise both arms until your palms face the wall behind you. Reach and hold for ten seconds. Return slowly to the starting position. Repeat four times.

30. *Hand Raiser*—Sit on a bench or stool with your back against the wall. Keep the arms straight and raise them sideward to shoulder height. Flex the elbows to 90° angles, with palms facing downward toward the floor. Slowly rotate the upper arms and lift the hands to touch the wall with the backs of the hands. Hold for four seconds; then slowly rotate the upper arms in the opposite direction and lower the hands to touch the wall with the palms. Hold for four seconds; slowly return the hands to shoulder height. Keep the elbows at shoulder height and at 90° angles throughout the movement. Relax and repeat four times.

31. *Hand-on-elbow Pull*—Sit or stand erect. Reach over your right shoulder with your right hand and place your fingers on the spine below shoulder height. Reach over your head with your left hand, grasp your right elbow, and slowly pull it down sliding the fingers down the center of your back. Hold for 20 seconds and then relax. Repeat four times and then change to the left side.

32. *Shoulder Stretch*—Tailor sit or stand. Reach the right hand over the right shoulder and down the spine and the left hand up your spine, and try to hook the fingers. Reverse, reaching with the left hand over the left shoulder and the right hand behind your back. Repeat four times.

33. *Inverted-T*—Assume a hook-lying position. Place the hands (palms up) on the floor and the elbows (flexed at a 90° angle) at shoulder height. Keep the backs of the hands and the elbows on the floor while slowly sliding the arms down until the elbows touch your rib cage. Repeat four times.

Flexibility: Waist and Trunk

34. *Lateral Stretch*—Stand in a side-stride position. Raise your right arm overhead, and lean to the left as you reach across the front of your body with your left arm. "Reach" in opposite directions four times. Alternate with the right side.

35. *Torso Twist*—Stand in a side-stride position, with your arms raised to the side at shoulder level. Keep your hips facing forward, as your upper trunk and head "twist" to the left until your right arm is extended forward and your left arm is extended backward. Return to the starting position, and then twist to the right side. Your eyes should follow the hand that is behind you. Repeat four sets.

36. *Body Bender*—Stand in a side-stride position, with the hands behind your neck and the fingers interlaced. Bend the trunk *sideward* to the left as far as possible; return to the starting position; bend the trunk *sideward* to the right. Repeat four sets.

37. *Knee Over*—Lie supine with the legs extended, arms at the sides. Slide the right foot up until the lower leg is perpendicular to the floor. Keeping your shoulders in contact with the floor, try to touch the floor beside your left hip with your right knee. Return to the initial position and repeat with the left knee. Alternating legs, repeat six sets.

Flexibility: Lower Back and Legs

(See pages 132 and 133.)

38. *Hamstring Stretch*—Sit on floor with legs extended. Bend your right knee and rest the sole of the right foot against the inside left thigh. Lean forward and grasp the ankle of the left foot with both hands. Hold an easy stretch for 20 to 40 seconds. Relax, then repeat. Repeat actions with other leg.

39. *Back Stretch*—Lie on your back with the legs extended. Bend your right leg and grasp the right thigh with hands and pull to chest; return to the starting position and repeat four times. Repeat pulling the left thigh.

40. *Knee-to-Nose Extension*—On hands and knees, bring your right knee to your nose, and then extend the leg out backwards as you lift your head. Repeat four times, and then change to the left leg. Repeat four sets. (Caution: do not raise the leg above the horizontal or arch your back or neck.)

41. *Sprinter's Crouch*—Squat, place the hands on the floor in line with the shoulders, and point the fingers forward. Extend the left leg fully to the rear. Slowly lower the left hip down and up four times; reverse the legs, and repeat with the right leg extended. Repeat four sets.

42. *"Gastroc" Stretch*—Stand in a lunge position, left foot forward and right foot back, with trunk erect and hands on left thigh. Keep the toes of both feet pointing forward and the heels in contact with the floor. Move your right foot back until you feel your calf muscles stretch. Keep your knee straight and heel on the floor. Hold an easy stretch for 20 to 40 seconds. Relax; repeat action. Repeat actions with the right foot forward.

43. *"Soleus" Stretch*—Same as number 42 except slowly bend your back knee while keeping your back heel on the floor. You should feel a stretch in the Achilles tendon.

44. *Quadricep Stretch*—Sit on the floor with your left leg extended, bend your right leg, and place the right foot flat on the floor to the left of the left knee. Turn your head and trunk to the right, place your right hand on the floor behind you, and place your left elbow against the right side of the right knee. Try to look behind you over your right shoulder. Hold for 20 to 40 seconds. Repeat with your right leg extended and head and trunk turned to the left.

SELECTED EXERCISES FOR FIGURE/PHYSIQUE IMPROVEMENT

Bust/Chest

The breasts are glands, not muscles; therefore, exercises for the bust are of doubtful value. However, exercises which improve the strength of the chest muscles (pectorals) supporting the bust, combined with good posture can help a woman appear well endowed. Strangely enough, the same exercise may help decrease the measurements of those who are overendowed, but you should be realistic in your expectations; exercises will not make the big person small nor the small, big. Men should use the same exercises to improve their posture and physique.

Push-ups—See page 60, exercise 11.
Arm Circles—See page 79, exercise 4.
Bench Press—See page 54, exercise 3.

45. *Isometric Push-Pull*—Sit or stand. Hold your arms in front of you at shoulder height and flex your elbows. Grasp your right wrist with your left hand and your left wrist with your right hand. Push strongly toward your elbows, then try to pull your hands apart. Feel the chest muscles contracting as you push and the upper back muscles contract as you pull.

Waist

The front half of your waist is made up of the abdominal muscles so abdominal strengthening exercises, such as isometrics and crunches, are the most effective waist exercises. To develop all of the muscles, however, execute your crunches with a twist to the right and left. These same exercises will help rid you of abdominal ptosis. An exercise to help strengthen the side and back muscles (at the same time they are increasing flexibility), consists of holding a weight in one hand and bending the trunk sideward in the opposite direction. (See page 58, exercise 7.) If your waist is big because of fat, these local exercises will not reduce the fat. Men tend to deposit fat here and develop a "pot."

Hips

To firm flabby hip muscles, you need to perform strength and endurance exercises for the buttocks muscles ("gluts") which cross the hip joint at the back. (See page 61.) Also, this can be accomplished by simply contracting the "seat" muscles isometrically. Other appropriate exercises include back exercises in chapter 9, knee-to-nose extension (page 64, exercise 40), and half-squats (page 56, exercise 5).

For most women it is the padding (sometimes known as "saddlebags") on the sides of the hips that is of the most concern. Just remember that it is the "nature of the female species" to have a broad pelvis and fat deposits on the hips and thighs. Strengthening the gluteus muscles and other muscles that cross the side of the hip joint will help tighten the flab but not the fat in that region. *Side leg raises* (see XBX exercise 7a) are useful for this purpose, as are *isometric contractions. Running, rope jumping, stair climbing,* and *jumping jacks* also employ the hip muscles.

Calf

Men, more than women sometimes want to develop a larger calf muscle. *Running* and *jumping* help, but, more specifically, exercises which cause toe-pointing against resistance will strengthen the calf muscle. *Tip-toeing* with weights on the shoulders or in the hands is one example. (See page 57, exercise 6.)

Thighs

Hip exercises are useful for strengthening (and therefore, firming) the thighs. Half-knee squats (page 56, exercise 5) are good for this. *Knee extensions* on a weight training machine will develop the quadriceps as will exercises 22–26 on page 62.

46. Another exercise you may wish to add is *leg circling*. Lie supine and raise one leg to make a 90° angle with the hip (avoid arching the back). Move it in clockwise and counterclockwise circles, or write your name and address in the air. Keep your leg straight; make the movement from the hip joint. This is more effective if ankle weights are used.

The muscles on the inside of the thigh, the adductors, are particularly prone to flabbiness because they are rarely used vigorously in everyday activity. *Horseback riding* and *swimming the breaststroke* bring them into play, but these sports are not enjoyed by all. Specifically for that region, try an isometric contraction by sitting on the floor and placing your feet on the outside of a chair. *Squeeze*—try to push the chair legs together. Or sit facing a partner in stride position and try to push their legs together. A *side-lying leg lift* using the bottom leg rather than the top is effective, especially with ankle weights added.

Upper Arms

For those of you who want better muscle definition or who wish to get rid of flabby arms and increase strength, the *triceps curl* (elbow extension) or the *biceps curl* (elbow flexion) against resistance are the most popular exercises. See pages 53–54, exercises 1–4, and exercises 9–14 on page 80.

REFERENCES

1. "News You Can Use In Your Personal Planning," *U.S. News & World Report,* (May 1, 1978):93.
2. Harris, G. and Gurin, J. "Look Who's Getting It All Together," *American Health,* (March, 1985):42–47.
3. Pollock, M. "How Much Exercise Is Enough?" in D. E. Cundiff (Ed.), *Implementation of Health Fitness Exercise Programs,* Reston, VA: American Alliance for Health, Physical Education, Recreation and Dance, 1985, pp. 59–69.
4. Cooper, K. H. *The Aerobics Way.* New York: M. Evans and Company, Inc., 1977, pp. 280–281.
5. Rogers, C. C. "On the Rebound: A Fitness Love Affair," *Physician and Sports Medicine,* (Sept. 1985): 141–150.
6. Griffith, B. R. and Martin, P. "Ballroom Aerobics," *Dance Magazine,* (Dec. 1985):99.
7. Cooper, *The Aerobics Way,* 1977, pp. 79–80.
8. Cooper, K. H. *Running Without Fear,* New York: Bantam Books, 1985, pp. 114–131.
9. Parry, A. "The Workout of the Future," *Shape,* (Sept. 1987):106.

Fitness Programs

5

PRETEST

1. How are training programs designed to accommodate a variety of interests, skill, and fitness levels?
2. How does one increase the level of intensity of a workout?
3. What role can sports and games play in a fitness training program?
4. What are some predesigned training programs that are available?

Getting in shape, and staying that way, appears to be relatively easy for some people; but, for others, it seems to be an almost insurmountable, and never ending task. You must do physical work to "get in shape," therefore, it will be to your advantage to select and incorporate into a program activities that you enjoy doing, are capable of performing, are not dangerous to your health, and are accessible. The programs described in this chapter may serve as beginning ones for many of you and as a base for others who wish to eventually design their own. Remember that no one program is appropriate for all; modifications in the design may be necessary for some individuals.

WALKING

You should have little difficulty following this program as walking is a locomotor movement that most of you already do at various times throughout the day. A sample training program is shown in Table IX. Stay on one step until you have walked the distance in the suggested time at least three times. If you are walking slowly, the walk itself serves as a warm-up and cool-down; however, if you are walking at a brisk pace, you should take the time to warm-up before and cool-down after the walk.

TABLE IX
Walking Program

Step 1. Prepare

    a. Get a log book for recording times and distances and a good pair of walking shoes.

    b. Measure a course in increments of one-fourth miles.

    c. Establish short range and long range goals.

Step 2. Begin to walk. Walk easily and do not be concerned with time or distance; stop when you wish.

Step 3. Walk one mile.

Step 4. Walk one mile in 15 minutes.

Step 5. Walk two miles.

Step 6. Walk two miles in 30 minutes.

Step 7. Walk three miles.

Step 8. Walk three miles in 45 minutes.

Step 9. Walk three miles in 45 minutes and carry very light (one pound) handweights.

JOGGING

The program shown in Table X is for beginners. You "aim" to continue to increase your jogging time as you work within your limits and toward personal objectives. Work toward advancing a level each week, but progress only when you can jog and talk at the same time. Jog on alternate days to give your body time to recover.

ROPE JUMPING

Before beginning to jump, stretch and warm-up with a variety of low-intensity exercises; pay special attention to the calf muscles and to the quadriceps. At the end of the work-out, cool down, giving special consideration to the primary muscles involved in performing this exercise. Rope jumping can be a very intense exercise and should not be attempted by everyone. If there is a question about your health status, check with your physician before beginning this, or any, potentially physically demanding activity. A sample program is shown in Table XI. Jump with both feet simultaneously and be sure to remain on each step until you can perform the routine comfortably.

TABLE X
Introduction to Jogging

Level	Routine	Repetitions	Total Time* (min.)	Jogging Time (min.)
1	Walk Briskly 2 min. Jog 1 min.	6	18	6
2	Walk briskly 90 sec. Jog 90 sec.	6	18	9
3	Walk briskly 1 min. Jog 2 min.	6	18	12
4	Walk briskly 1 min. Jog 3 min.	5	20	15
5	Walk briskly 1 min. Jog 4 min.	4	20	16
6	Walk briskly 1 min. Jog 5 min. Then walk 1 min., jog 2	3 1	21	17
7	Walk briskly 1 min. Jog 6 min.	3	21	18
8	Walk briskly 1 min. Jog 7 min. Then walk 1 min., jog 5	2 1	22	19

*Total time exclusive of warm-up and cool-down.

TABLE XI
Rope Jumping Program

Step 1. Jump 50 times without pausing at the rate of 90 jumps per minute. If you miss, begin counting at 0; continue trying until you have reached the magic number of 50. You may find that this goal is a bit high for you; if so, set a lower number.

Step 2. Keep jumping until you can jump 100 times without missing and when you can do this, jump 100 times, walk for 30 seconds, jump another 100 times, and walk again. Adapt to this level.

Step 3. Jump three sets of 100 jumps. Walk for 30 seconds between sets. Adapt to this level.

Step 4. Jump for time—try for six to eight consecutive minutes at the beginning. Gradually increase the time until you can jump for 15 consecutive minutes. Adapt to this level.

Step 5. Use a weighted rope (two pounds for beginners) to increase upper body strength and aerobic capacity.

SWIMMING (continuously)

Swim continuously, using any stroke but preferably the overhand crawl, for 30 minutes. It may help you to maintain your swimming pace for this length of time if you wear a mask and use a snorkel. Some may find that wearing swim fins is advantageous. Increase the level of intensity of the continuous swim by using the crawl stroke for longer periods of time.

INTERVAL TRAINING

Interval Rope Jumping Program

Take precautions as you would for any potentially strenuous activity before beginning this type of program. Warm-up and cool-down as you would for any activity; pay particular attention to the muscle groups that are involved in jumping. Jump for 60 seconds, walk for 60 seconds, and continue this pattern for 20 to 25 minutes.

Interval Swimming Program

If you choose to work out every other day, select either continuous swimming (above) or interval swimming. If you are working-out every day, alternate between the two. After you can perform at these beginning levels of the interval program comfortably, increase the work part in increments of 25 yards.

TABLE XII
Starter Interval Swimming Program

Step 1.	Use the overhand crawl stroke to swim 25 to 100 yards (depending upon your fitness and/or skill level) without pausing.
Step 2.	Follow this with a resting stroke or walk in the water until your breathing rate returns to normal.
Step 3.	Repeat the crawl stroke, follow with the resting stroke or walk in the water, and continue this pattern until you have worked out for 30 minutes.

ACCELERATED CYCLING

Table XIII outlines an acceleration cycling (stationary bicycle) training program in which the speed (miles per hour which can be easily read on the odometer) of pedaling varies among intervals. The intensity can be modified to meet individual needs by increasing or decreasing speeds, pedal resistance, or the number of sets; you must work above your threshold level. However, the basic format of gradually increasing speed (accelerating) and maintaining a balance between rest and work should remain. Remember to include warm up and cool down periods.

TABLE XIII
Introduction to Accelerated Cycling

Set	Intensity (mph)	Duration (min.)
1	Resting pace	3
	5	1
	10	1
	15	1
2	Resting pace	3
	5	1
	10	1
	15	1
3	Resting pace	3
	5	1
	10	1
	15	1
4	Resting pace	3
	5	1
	10	1
	15	1
5	Resting pace	3
	5	1
	10	1
	15	1

AEROBIC DANCE ROUTINE*

Remember to follow the general guidelines for exercising as well as those that apply specifically to an aerobic dance workout. These include:

1. Wear good aerobic shoes.
2. Know your limits and listen to your body; do not over-stretch or perform a high-impact routine when you are not ready for it.

*Used by permission of Renee-Patin Fry. Community Health and Wellness Graduate. Oklahoma State University.

3. Avoid twisting hop variations that place undue stress on your spine.
4. Make sure that your heels go all the way to the floor when you do high-impact exercises.
5. Limit your hopping on one foot to a maximum of four consecutive times.
6. Do low-impact exercises before and after doing high-impact ones—work "into" and "out of" a strenuous routine.

Phase One: Warm-up

This phase should last at least five minutes to prepare the body for aerobic exercise. Warming up will gradually increase the heart rate, acquaint the body with a new workload, and minimize the risk of musculoskeletal injury. This is a great time to perform exercises that will enhance flexibility, muscular strength, and muscular endurance. The following warm-up will provide adequate stretching exercises to precede the aerobic activity:

Toe Raises—Lift and lower your heels for 20 counts to increase blood circulation and help warm up the legs.

Shoulder Circles—Circle the shoulders forward and backward (each direction, eight counts) to stretch shoulders and surrounding muscles. (You may choose to only circle backward because too many individuals have "round shoulders.")

Side Stretches—With both arms directly overhead, stretch to the right and hold for eight counts. Remember to go to the side (not front or back) with the abdomen pulled in as tight as possible. Do the same for the left side.

Front Stretch—Once again, arms are directly overhead, knees are slightly bent, and feet are shoulder distance apart. Bend at the waist and reach forward to stretch the hamstrings and lower back muscles. Hold for eight counts.

Toe Stretch—From the previous position, reach down toward the floor to stretch the back, hamstrings, calves, and gluteal muscles. Knees are still slightly bent and feet are shoulder distance apart. Hold the position for eight counts.

Toe Raises—Now walk your hands forward on the floor away from your feet to assume a comfortable position. Lift and lower your heels. When lifting the heel, raise it as high as possible over your toes; likewise, when lowering your heels, lower them completely to the floor. Do this for eight counts to stretch the calves.

Calf Stretches—Press both heels simultaneously to the floor and hold for eight counts. Hands are still forward on the floor away from the feet. Stretching the calves a great deal because they will work frequently during the aerobic activity.

Single Calf Stretches—From the previous position, lift your left foot in the air while the right heel is completely on the floor. Hold for eight counts. Repeat this exercise for the left calf. (Walk your hands back to the feet. Feet are still shoulder distance apart.)

Single Leg Stretches—Press the torso of the body toward the right leg. Knees are slightly bent, and the chest should press toward the right knee. Hold for eight counts and do the same for the left leg to stretch the hamstrings of both legs.

Lunge Stretch—Stand with feet together and hands to your sides. Step forward with the right leg to a bent knee position. Keep the back leg extended, allowing it to bend slightly. Make sure not to stretch with the right knee protruding past the right foot. Support your weight by placing your hands on either side of the body on the floor. Hold this position for eight counts while stretching the quadriceps and hamstrings. Reverse legs and stretch with the left leg in front.

Inner Thigh Stretches—Sit on the floor and pull feet into the groin with hands, push knees down to the floor. Bend forward with upper torso to achieve a better stretch. Make sure the inside of the knees are facing up toward the ceiling. Hold for eight counts. (Slowly release from the stretch and stand to prepare for the aerobic activity.)

Phase Two: Low-Impact Aerobics

This phase should be done for a *minimum* of 20 minutes, at least three times a week. Start off with some low-impact exercises to increase the heart rate to its target level gradually. The following lists will provide you with some leg movements and arm movements that you can put together in any combination. Choose any of these exercises in any order; it does not matter what you do, as long as you keep moving! Do the low-impact activity for at least five minutes before attempting high-impact. You could fill the entire aerobic activity time with lower-impact exercise to minimize the stress on the joints that accompanies high-impact aerobics.

Leg Movements

Walk in place

Knee lifts in place

Side Steppers—Step from side to side.

Step Kicks—Step with one foot and kick with the other; alternate.

Knee Bends—With feet shoulder distance apart, bend knees like you are about to sit in a chair. Bend and stand to the beat.

Arm Movements

Scissors—Scissor the arms out in front, behind your back, or overhead for variation.

Row-pulls—Arms are to the sides. Pull elbows directly upward and release.

Bicep Curls—Arms are horizontally out to the sides. Elbows should remain shoulder height during this exercise. Curl arms in by bending at the elbow, then straighten.

Tricep Curls—Arms are once again horizontally extended out to the sides. Keep those elbows shoulder height. Bend at the elbows and curl inward in a pendulum motion, then straighten.

Good-byes—Arms are directly overhead. Wave to the right then left with the arms in waving motion together.

Phase Three: High-Impact Aerobics

This is the high intensity phase of the routine. If you cannot talk "normally" while doing these exercises, you are probably attempting to work at a level that is too high for you.

Leg Movements

Jog in place

Power Knees—Jog in place lifting each knee as high as possible.

Jump Ropes—Use an imaginary rope to jump.

Cross Country—Act as if you were skiing cross-country.

Ski Hops—Hop from side to side as if you were going over moguls.

Jumping Jacks

Jumping Jacks with Criss-Cross—Do normal jumping jacks but as feet come together, cross them in the middle.

Knee Lifts with Hops

Jump Kicks—Jump with both feet and kick to the side with one foot. Then, jump with feet together and kick with the other foot.

Arm Movements

Do any of the arm movements previously discussed while jogging in place.

Phase Four: Low-Impact Aerobics

Do low-impact aerobics for at least five minutes to reduce the heart rate to a normal level. See exercises listed Phase Two of the routine.

Phase Five: Cool-Down

Restretch the muscles by doing the warm-up phase in reverse. Finish off with some deep breathing to get oxygen to the brain.

TABLE XIV
Continuous Exercise Routine (could be set to music)

Exercise	Time (min.)	Activity	Description
1	1	Shoulder Stretch	See page 63, Exercise 32
2	1	Gastroc Stretch	See page 64, Exercise 42
3	1	Step and Reach	Stand with arms at sides. Take a long step forward with right foot and reach forward with arms; repeat with left foot. Step to the side with the right foot and raise the arms sideward; repeat with left foot. Step backwards with the right foot and reach the arms backwards; repeat with left foot. Repeat as time permits.
4	1	Overhead Reach/ Toe Touch	Stand on tiptoes and reach high 5 times; touch fingers to toes or floor 5 times. (Repeat if time permits.)
5	2	Walk/Jog	Walk 2 gym laps; jog 2 laps. Breathe deeply; swing arms briskly. (Repeat if time permits.)
6	1	Push-ups	See pages 4 and 60, Exercise 11
7	½	Arm Backs	See page 62, Exercise 27
8	½	Jumping Jacks	
9	1	Roll Downs	See page 61, Exercise 15
10	3	Walk/Skip/Gallop	Walk 1 lap at a fast pace; skip 1 lap; gallop 1 lap (Repeat if time permits.)
11	1	High Stepper	Stand erect with elbows bent and hands relaxed. Walk in place; lift feet about a foot off the floor and pump arms vigorously.
12	½	Foot Circling	See page 113, Exercise 7
13	½	Knee-to-Nose Extension	See page 64, Exercise 40
14	3	Jog	Jog at medium pace.
15	2	Walk	Walk at medium pace. Breathe deeply; swing arms briskly.
16	1	Sprinter's Crouch	See page 64, Exercise 41
17	1	Knee Raise	See page 79, Exercise 2
18	1	Mad Cat	See page 151, Exercise 0
19	1	Quad Stretch	See page 64, Exercise 44

CONTINUOUS EXERCISE

It should be relatively easy for you to design a continuous exercise routine that will allow you to meet your personal needs and interests. The one shown in Table XIV is representative of what can be done by following the suggestions for exercising found in chapter 3.

XBX EXERCISE PLAN

The Royal Canadian Air Force (RCAF) designed an exercise plan for women, called the "XBX."[1] It is suitable for men and women, but men may be able to progress faster. The plan consists of four charts of 10 exercises each arranged in progressive order of difficulty. Each chart is divided into 12 performance levels, numbered consecutively from one (the easiest) to 48 (the most difficult). A total of 12 minutes is allowed in which to perform the entire routine, and there is a time limit for each exercise; however, you may choose to forget the time and concentrate on doing the exercises correctly and for the predetermined number of times. The number of repetitions of each exercise increases as you advance to higher levels, and the exercises are modified to become more difficult as you move to the next higher chart. Do not skip levels as you progress. A healthy young adult should spend at least one day at each level on Chart I, two days at each level on Chart II. Move to a new level when you can perform the routine without undue strain or soreness. When you have reached your maximum level of performance, three exercise periods per week should be adequate to maintain it. Only two levels are included in the book because if you can perform at this level, you are probably ready for a more advanced program.

As with all exercise workouts, you should do cool-down exercises after completing the XBX routine. Walking and stretching exercises are useful for this purpose. The exercises are designed to use most of the major muscle groups of the body, and to develop the health related physical fitness components. The primary purposes of each of the exercises are described below.

Purpose of each XBX Exercise

1. *Toe Touch*—Flexibility; stretches muscles in lower back and in back of legs.
2. *Knee Raise*—Flexibility; stretches lower back and hip muscles, and helps improve endurance and strength of muscles on the front of the thighs (good for lordosis).
3. *Lateral Bend*—Flexibility and endurance and strength of trunk muscles.
4. *Arm Circle*—Flexibility; stretches pectoral muscle across chest; also increases endurance and strength of muscles in the upper back. (Good for round shoulders, kyphosis, and sunken chest.)

5. *Sit-ups*—Strengthens abdominals.
6. a. *Chest and Leg Raise*—Increases endurance and strength of back and hip muscles. (Good for kyphosis).
   b. *Knee-to-Nose Touch*—Stretches lower back; improves endurance and strength of upper back and hip muscles.
7. a. *Side Leg Raise*—Increases endurance and strength of muscles on side of hip and thigh.
   b. *Leg Over*—Strengthens trunk muscles as well as thigh muscles.
8. *Push-ups*—Increases endurance and strength of chest muscles and back of upper arms.
9. *Leg Lift*—Increases endurance and strength of muscles on front of thigh.
10. *Run and Hop, Run-and-Stride Jump*—Cardiovascular endurance; increases strength and endurance of muscles in legs and hips.

TABLE XV
Chart I of the XBX Program

Level	Exercise									
	1	2	3	4	5	6	7	8	9	10
12	9	8	10	40	26	20	28	14	14	170
11	9	8	10	40	24	18	26	13	14	160
10	9	8	10	40	22	16	25	12	12	150
9	7	7	8	36	20	14	23	10	11	140
8	7	7	8	36	18	12	20	9	10	125
7	7	7	8	36	16	12	18	8	10	115
6	5	5	7	28	14	10	16	7	8	100
5	5	5	7	28	12	8	13	6	6	90
4	5	5	7	28	10	8	10	5	6	80
3	3	4	5	24	8	6	8	4	4	70
2	3	4	5	24	6	4	6	3	3	60
1	3	4	5	24	4	4	4	3	2	50
Minutes for each exercise	2	2	2	2	2	1	1	2	1	3

Chart I Exercises

1. a. **Toe Touch.** Feet 12″ apart; arms overhead; try to touch toes. Do not lock your knees.
   b. **Alternate.*** Same as above, except perform in sitting position.
2. **Knee Raise.** Raise alternate knees and pull thigh toward chest with hands; keep back straight; left plus right is 1 count.
3. **Lateral Bend.** Feet 12″ apart; alternate sideward, bending to right and left, sliding hand down leg as far as possible; left plus right is 1 count.
4. **Arm Circle.*** Feet 12″ apart; make large backward circles with arms; alternating right, left, right, etc. Keep palms of hands facing upward.
5. **Partial Sit-ups.** Back lying; arms at side; raise head and shoulders until you can see your heels.
6. a. **Chest and Leg Raise.** Front lying; hands under thighs; raise head and shoulders and alternate legs as high as possible; left is one count, right is one count.
   b. **Knee-to-Nose Touch.*** (For those with lordosis.) On hands and knees, try to touch nose with knee; then extend leg backward *parallel* with floor while raising head; do not arch back; half of repetitions with right leg, half with left.
7. **Side Leg Raise.** Side lying; use arms for balance; raise upper leg 18–24 inches; half of repetitions left leg, half right.
8. **Push-ups.** Front lying; hands under shoulders; push up and rock back on heels; keep hands and knees on floor; return to starting position.
9. **Leg Lift.** Back lying; arms at side; raise alternate legs perpendicular to floor; left plus right is 1 count.
10. **Run and Hop.** Run in place; lift knees and feet at least 4″ high; left plus right is 1 count; after 50 counts, jump up and down 10 times, lifting feet at least 4″ high.

Chart II Exercises

(Same as Chart I, except as noted.)

1. **Toe Touch.***
   a. Bend slowly, touching floor at heel level.
   b. Alternate.* Same as in Chart I.
2. **Knee Raise.** Same as in Chart I.
3. **Lateral Bend.*** Same as Chart I.
4. **Arm Circle.*** Circle both arms backward simultaneously. Keep palms facing up.
5. **Rocking Sit-ups.** Back lying with knees bent; arms overhead; swing arms and sit up while legs extend; try to touch toes; return to starting position.

* Starred exercises are those revised by the authors.
Those persons with lordosis should perform exercise 6.b. rather than 6.a.

TABLE XVI
Chart II of the XBX Program

Level	Exercise									
	1	**2**	**3**	**4**	**5**	**6**	**7**	**8**	**9**	**10**
24	15	16	12	30	35	38	50	28	20	210
23	15	16	12	30	33	36	48	26	18	200
22	15	16	12	30	31	34	48	24	18	200
21	13	14	11	26	29	32	44	23	16	190
20	13	14	11	26	27	31	42	21	16	175
19	13	14	11	26	24	29	40	20	14	160
18	12	12	9	20	22	27	38	18	14	150
17	12	12	9	20	19	24	36	16	12	150
16	12	12	9	20	16	21	34	14	10	140
15	10	10	7	18	14	18	32	14	10	130
14	10	10	7	18	11	15	30	10	8	120
13	10	10	7	18	9	12	28	8	8	120
Minutes for each exercise	2½	2½	2½	2½	2½	1	1	2½	1	3

6. a. **Chest and Leg Raise.** Lift head and shoulders and both legs at same time. Do not arch your lower back.
   b. **Knee-to-Nose Touch.*** Same as in Chart I.
7. **Side Leg Raise.*** Try to raise leg to a 45° angle. Be sure that it is sideward, not forward.
8. a. **Knee Push-ups.** Keep body line straight while pushing up and down; do not rock back on heels.
   b. **Alternate.*** Lean against a low bench and push up.
9. **Leg Overs.** Back lying; arms out at shoulder level; raise one leg to perpendicular and try to touch opposite hand with toes; return to perpendicular and to starting position; alternate legs; left is 1 count; right is 1 count.
10. **Run-and-Stride Jump.** Do 10 jumping-jacks after every 50 runs.

* Starred exercises are those revised by the authors.
Those persons with lordosis should perform exercise 6.b. rather than 6.a.

HEALTH RELATED FITNESS BENEFITS OF SELECTED SPORTS

Some of you may prefer to participate in a sport or game rather than to do calisthenic-type exercises. As is true for any physical activity, the benefits derived are dependent upon how often you play, how hard you play, and how long you play. For many of you, it may be best to get into shape first and then select a sport to play. The better choices are those that are rhythmic in nature, require you to use large muscle groups, and allow you to sustain an elevated heart rate. Table XVII, showing ratings of selected sports on a scale of one (low) to four (high), can be used as a guide to help you design a training program if playing a sport is to be your primary means of developing fitness or maintaining it.

TABLE XVII
Fitness Ratings of Sports

Sport	Cardiovascular Endurance	Strength	Muscular Endurance	Flexibility	Body Composition
Archery	1	2	1	1	1
Badminton	3	1	2	2	3
Basketball	4	1	2	1	3
Bowling	1	1	1	1	1
Football	2	3	2	1	2
Golf (walking)	2	1	1	2	2
Gymnastics	2	4	4	4	2
Handball	3	1	3	1	3
Karate	1	2	2	2	1
Racketball	3	1	3	1	3
Soccer	4	2	3	2	3
Slowpitch Softball	1	1	1	1	2
Table Tennis	1	1	1	1	1
Tennis	2	1	2	1	2
Ultimate Frisbee	3	1	2	3	3
Volleyball	2	2	1	1	1

REFERENCE

1. Royal Canadian Air Force, *Royal Canadian Air Force Exercise Plans for Physical Fitness* (Ottawa, Canada: Queen's Printer). Used by special arrangement with *This Week Magazine* (New York: United Newspapers Magazine Corp).

Weight, Fatness, and Nutrition

6

PRETEST

1. Why is it important to maintain proper weight?
2. What are anorexia nervosa and bulemia?
3. What causes obesity?
4. What is a balanced diet?
5. How many calories per day do you need?
6. How useful is exercise in a weight control program?

America has a greater abundance of food than any other country in the world—it is also more highly mechanized, with labor saving devices which decrease the need for energy expenditure. Is it any wonder that half of our population is overfat, and that eating and dieting are adult preoccupations? Engineers have calculated that if all of that excess fat were converted to an equal quantity of fuel oil, it would supply the electrical needs of Orange County, California for at least 100 days!

BODY COMPOSITION

Many people, especially teenagers and young adults, are dissatisfied with their estimated "ideal" weight and feel that they should weigh much less because they want smaller girth measurements. This is usually due to a misconception about body composition and confusion of the terms *weight* and *fatness*. Your fatness is a more important indication of health (and appearance) than your weight. Most people need to strive for *leanness,* not lightness! It is possible to reduce girth measurements by losing fat and increasing muscle, without changing weight; sometimes one can lose inches and even experience a weight gain!

The percentage of fat in the body can be estimated indirectly by several sophisticated laboratory procedures, such as hydrostatic (underwater) weighing, total body counters, neutron activation analysis, CAT scans, and others. There are also some relatively simple techniques, such as skinfold measures. Approximately 50 percent of our total body fat lies just under the skin and can be pinched-up and measured by skin calipers. By measuring several predetermined sites on the body and computing by formulae, a fairly accurate assessment of the relative leanness-fatness composition of the body may be made.

All techniques are only estimates and even the most sophisticated procedures have three to four percent error. Simpler methods have even more error and for that reason, if possible, it is best to use more than one technique for estimating body composition. It is also important that tables which prescribe desirable standards such as those in chapter 1 give ranges rather than single numbers because the norms are based on averages and any one individual may deviate considerably from the average.

DESIRABLE BODY WEIGHT

"Desirable" or "ideal" body weight differs greatly among individuals—even individuals of the same age and height will not necessarily have the same "ideal" weight, because of differences in skeletal size, bone density, and muscle mass. However, your weight should be within approximately 10 percent of your estimated "ideal" weight range. If you are more than 10 percent above or below this figure, you may be considered overweight or underweight, respectively. (If you are 20 percent over the "ideal," you are classified as obese.) The "ideal" weight may be modified to some extent by heavy musculature; therefore, an individual may be overweight without being overfat. Some athletes may be classified as overweight, yet they may not have an ounce of surplus fat on them. On the other hand, some sedentary individuals may be overfat (fat weighs less than muscle) without being overweight.

Desirable or ideal body weight is hard to define because there is no sound scientific evidence which allows us to compute how much any one individual should weigh. Furthermore, what one might consider an "ideal" weight for health might not be "ideal" for appearance; and what is "ideal" for appearance might not be "ideal" for performance. Nevertheless, there are at least two good reasons for being concerned about weight. One is that it is easy to step onto a set of scales and measure your weight and most people have access to scales whereas they may not have access to the more sophisticated equipment and the expertise needed for measuring body composition. Secondly, insurance companies and researchers from the Framingham Heart Study have found overweight to be a health hazard. And the 1985 National Institutes of Health (NIH) Consensus Conference on Obesity concluded that a level of 20 percent or more above "desirable" weight is the point where physicians should treat an otherwise healthy person.[1] Dr. Jules Hirsch, chairman of that 14 member panel of experts indicated that risks to health occur at even five to

10 pounds above desirable weight.[2] The standard used by the Consensus Conference is the Metropolitan Insurance Company height-weight chart included in chapter 1. (Many experts feel that these weights are slightly high since they are based on average weights of the population in the western world and that figure has increased over the past 40 years.)[3,4] Your frame (skeletal) size cannot be determined simply by measuring the wrist, or the elbow or the pelvic and shoulder widths but such a measurement may be of some assistance in helping you to estimate your skeletal size.

OTHER TECHNIQUES FOR SCREENING OBESITY

Abdominal vs Hip Girth

Several studies have indicated that the location of fat deposits may be a better predictor of coronary heart disease than the degree of obesity. Excess abdominal fat is more often related to disease than are fat deposits in the thigh or gluteal areas. The risk increases sharply when a man's waist measures the same as or bigger than his hip measurement. The same is true for a woman if her waist is **not** at least 20 percent smaller than her hips. (See chapter 1.)

Body Mass Index (BMI)

The NIH Consensus Development Conference recommended that health professionals utilize the BMI to screen adults (over the age of 20) for obesity. The BMI [body weight in kg divided by (height in cm)^2] has been shown to have a direct and continuous relationship to morbidity and mortality in studies of large populations. (See chapter 1.)

Relative Weight (RW)

Relative weight is also a widely used method of obesity screening. RW = measured weight divided by the mid-point of the medium frame desirable weight recommended in the 1983 Metropolitan Life Insurance Company tables. An RW of 20 percent or more above desirable weight is associated with sufficient health risk to justify clinical intervention.[3,4] (See chapter 1.)

If you combine the results of several screening techniques such as skinfold tests, girth, BMI, and RW, you will have a reasonably good estimate of your status. Because none is absolutely accurate enough to be used alone, several estimates should show enough agreement to guide you in planning your fitness and nutrition program.

WHY MAINTAIN PROPER WEIGHT AND BODY COMPOSITION

All of us are interested in appearance. We want to have a good figure/physique to look good in our clothes, and to be able to wear the latest fashions. While proper weight does not ensure good body proportions and good posture, it helps—and an attractive appearance helps increase self-confidence and poise.

More important than the psychological rewards are the physiological (health) benefits. Being lean means we are less susceptible to certain diseases and have a better chance to live longer.

Dangers of Obesity

Obesity increases one's susceptibility to a long list of health hazards including: respiratory difficulties; cardiac enlargement; congestive heart failure; high blood pressure; difficulties during anesthesia, surgery, pregnancy, and childbirth; varicose veins; osteoarthritis; and gallbladder disease, to name a few. It has been discovered that there is a greater risk of breast cancer in obese women and a poorer chance of recovery. In addition, social pressures may result in the development of neurosis, with an obsessive concern with body image, passivity, withdrawal, and expectation of rejection. The mortality rate for markedly overweight men is 79 percent greater than for those of average weight. For markedly overweight women, it is 61 percent greater. Moderate overweight increases the death rate for men and women to 42 percent greater than normal.

Dangers of Being too Thin

In the past, it was thought that it was healthy to be skinny and that underweight persons outlived us all. Some research studies have suggested that underweight people may have higher death rates than people whose weight is normal. This was especially true of those who were at least 20 percent underweight. The exact cause of this increased mortality is not known at this time and more research needs to be done.

A disease that afflicts more than 280,000 Americans, especially women between the ages of 12–25 is called *anorexia nervosa.* One out of 100 adolescent girls may be affected. Those who suffer from anorexia nervosa are committed to self-starvation and frenetic activity as part of a relentless pursuit of excessive thinness. More than 15 percent of them will die from the affliction. Psychological disturbances cause an abnormal desire to lose weight and also, excessive concern about personal appearance may lead to pathological fear of overeating or becoming fat. Anorexia nervosa patients may lose as much as 50 percent of their normal weight and develop severe signs of protein-calorie malnutrition, multiple vitamin deficiency, amenorrhea, dehydration, and electrolyte disturbances.

Bulemia, a medical term for gorging, is a related syndrome, but the symptoms are definitely different from anorexia nervosa. Bulemics eat excessively, feel guilty and then engage in self-induced vomiting and the taking of as many as 40–50 laxatives a day to purge themselves. It has been called a "binge-guilt-vomit-pleasure-hunger-binge cycle" and it may occur up to 15 times per day. Bulemics usually maintain normal weight but their physical and psychological health deteriorates and they risk esophageal irritation, intestinal bleeding, stomach rupture, and death. This syndrome may affect as many as one out of five young college women, and the number of reported incidences among older women is increasing.

Both bulemia and anorexia nervosa are difficult to diagnose because the victims usually deny and try to hide their behaviors. Treatment is even more difficult to accomplish effectively. Typically it involves individual psychotherapy, nutritional therapy, and family counseling, but it may take several years to bring about a cure from these compulsive behaviors. If you wish to know more about these syndromes, make use of the resources at the end of this chapter.

CAUSES OF WEIGHT AND FATNESS PROBLEMS

Obesity as defined by the NIH Consensus Development Panel on Obesity is "an excess of body fat frequently resulting in a significant impairment of health." They concluded that 20 percent or more above desirable body weight met that criteria. This corresponds to a Body Mass Index above 26.4 for men and 25.8 for women (see chapter 1). Sports medicine experts define obesity in terms of body composition and consider men to be obese when their fat levels are 25 percent or more and women to be obese at 30 percent or more. As discussed earlier, the over-fat person is usually (but not always) overweight and the overweight person is usually (but not always) overfat. Obesity is a complex medical problem with multiple causes, including over-eating for psychological reasons; poor eating habits because of family or cultural influences; and over-eating because of a lack of knowledge about calories. In rare instances, a person may over-eat because of diminished taste-bud discrimination. Only about five percent of the obese population suffer from metabolic disturbances which predispose them to accumulating fat. The causes and cures are far more complicated than can be discussed in these pages, but if you have a weight/fat problem that seems more complicated than a caloric imbalance, seek medical advice and/or consult a registered dietician.

Regardless of the underlying causes, the jokers are right when they say overweight is caused by two things, "chewing and swallowing." Overweight/overfat is the result of consuming more calories than are burned. Maintaining proper weight is a matter of balancing input (calories) with output (activity). If the number of calories eaten equals the number burned, weight remains the same. When input exceeds output, weight is gained and deposited in the form of adipose tissue (fat). The distribution of this extra padding is controlled genetically and hormonally. Usually such tissue accumulates around the hips and thighs on women. Men tend to deposit it around the waist.

Underweight is ultimately the result of consuming fewer calories than are burned, but it is probably an equally complex medical problem. Often it is accompanied by high metabolic levels; nervousness, hyperactivity, or poor eating habits may play a role; abnormal food absorption or loss of calories through urine (as in diabetes) occur in rare cases; sometimes it is an inherited somatotype.

THE IMPORTANCE OF GOOD NUTRITION

Weight and fatness control require good nutrition and proper exercise. First, we will examine the role of nutrition. You should make an evaluation of the type and amount of food you consume in order to determine whether it is serving your body's needs (see sample Charts IX and X in the Appendix). Before you read this chapter, test yourself on your knowledge of nutrition and weight control by taking the quiz on Chart VIII in the Appendix.

BALANCED DIET

The essential components in a balanced diet are vitamins, minerals, protein, fats and oils, carbohydrates, water, roughage, and calories. These are found in the four food groups recommended for the daily diet.

1. *Dairy Products* (*milk and cheese*)—two or more servings.
2. *Meat, Fish, and Eggs* (*protein group*)—two or more servings.
3. *Vegetables and Fruits*—four or more servings.
4. *Breads and Cereals* (*grain products*)—four or more servings.

It has been estimated that six out of ten youths between the ages of 13 and 19 are malnourished. This does not mean that they are underfed, but rather that they are not eating balanced diets. Teenagers have an affinity for pop, candy, and corn chips; but this puts their health in jeopardy, their complexion in a mess and their bodies in an unattractive shape.

The Food and Nutrition Board of the National Academy of Sciences recommends a daily dietary allowance for normal persons living in the United States under normal environmental stresses.[5] As an example, for a woman weighing 128 pounds, height 64″, age 18–35, it recommends 2,000 calories; protein 55 grams; calcium 0.8 grams; iron 8 milligrams; vitamin A 5,000 international units; thiamin 1.0 milligrams; riboflavin 1.5 milligrams; niacin 13 milligrams, and ascorbic acid 55 milligrams. For a man weighing 154 pounds, height 69″, age 18–35, it recommends 2,800 calories; protein 65 grams; calcium 0.8 grams; iron 10 milligrams; vitamin A 5,000 international units; thiamin 1.4 milligrams; riboflavin 1.7 milligrams; niacin 18 milligrams, and ascorbic acid 60 milligrams. The recommended daily dietary allowance will, in most cases, exceed the minimum daily requirement and if the nutrients mentioned here are taken care of, the 40 or so other less important ones will be, also.

Proteins build and repair the body and provide energy. Ten to 15 percent of the daily caloric requirement should be provided by protein; good sources include eggs, fish, meat, poultry and dairy products. Beans, peas, lentils, nuts, and seeds may be substituted often for these to help keep cholesterol low.

Carbohydrates furnish energy. The exact amount of carbohydrates needed in the daily diet is not known, however the National Research Council suggests that normal adults require about 500 carbohydrate calories daily; most people far exceed this amount. Carbohydrate food should be selected for its vitamin and mineral content as well as for its caloric content. Such foods are called complex carbohydrates and include fruits, starchy vegetables, and whole grain cereals.

Fats furnish energy and carry vitamins A, D, E, and K. Many nutritionists recommend that 25–30 percent of one's caloric intake should be composed of fats. The normal diet probably provides at least the minimum amount of fat from meat and vegetable sources. In fact, the average American consumes a diet of 40–45 percent fat. Saturated fat should be held to less than 10 percent; polyunsaturated fat and cholesterol intake should be 250–300 mg. per day.

Minerals such as calcium and iron build and repair the body and regulate its processes. Good sources of calcium include fish, cheese, eggs, poultry, milk, yogurt, fresh fruits, and whole grains. (See chapter 12 regarding calcium and osteoporosis.) Generous amounts of iron may be found in liver, green vegetables, egg yolk, turkey, beef, oysters, and clams. The American Heart Association recommends limiting egg yolks to three or less per week.

Vitamins A, B-complex (thiamin, riboflavin, and niacin), C, and D also regulate the body's processes. Good sources of vitamin A include liver, cheese, corn, egg yolk, broccoli, sunflower seeds, tomatoes, and peas. The vitamin B-complexes are most abundant in liver, kidneys, cheese, egg yolk, fish, poultry, yogurt, and whole grains. Foods generous in vitamin C include citrus fruits, cantaloupe, corn, green vegetables, tomatoes, peas, and potatoes. The sunshine vitamin-D, is prominent in milk, eggs, liver, fish, and oysters. (See chapter 7 regarding Fad diets.)

SEVEN DIETARY GUIDELINES

The following dietary guidelines for Americans will help you eat wisely for health maintenance and weight control. They are supported by such groups as the American Dietetic Association, Public Health Department, American Heart Association, American Diabetes Association and many others:

1. Eat a variety of foods.
2. Maintain ideal weight.
3. Limit fat, saturated fat, and cholesterol.
4. Eat foods with adequate starch and fiber.
5. Limit sugar.
6. Limit sodium.
7. If you drink alcohol, do so in moderation.

DETERMINATION OF CALORIC NEEDS

The number of calories needed to maintain proper weight is a very individual matter and depends upon a number of factors: (1) *size*—height, bone size, and muscle mass; (2) *basal metabolic rate*—the BMR is determined by glandular function, is higher in men than women, and decreases with age; (3) *age*—activity and metabolism decrease with age, so about 5 percent fewer calories are needed each 10 years after age 25 (the average age when growth ceases); (4) *activity*—the number of calories burned depends upon how many muscles are used; whether they are large or small muscles; how fast, how hard, and how long the activity is continued; (5) *climate*—more calories are burned in colder climate; (6) *timing of maturation*—early maturing women are fatter than late maturers; (7) *pregnancy and lactation*—may increase caloric needs, and (8) *temperament*—highstrung people burn more calories than relaxed people. The National Foods and Nutrition Board has made charts for estimating caloric needs based on these factors, but a quick method of estimating an individual's needs is based on the fact that the *average person needs about 15 calories per pound of body weight.* You can figure your approximate needs by multiplying 15 times your **optimum** weight to estimate what is required to maintain that weight. Keep in mind the eight factors mentioned previously, and remember it is only a crude estimate. The only satisfactory method of determining your need is to ascertain whether you are maintaining your optimum weight on that amount—if so, then that is the number of calories you need. If your weight is moving in the wrong direction, either your activity or both your activity and caloric input should be adjusted.

Strangely enough, more is known about weight loss than about weight gain. It is well established that regardless of how much one weighs, *a pound of fat will be lost for every 3,500 calorie deficit.* However, scientists do not clearly understand the mechanism (called **thermogenesis**) used to resist weight gain; thus it is not possible to predict the amount of weight you will gain on a given diet. According to Connor, "by current estimates, it may take from 500 to 5,000 calories or more to gain one pound."[6]

THE ROLE OF EXERCISE IN WEIGHT AND FAT LOSS

To lose a pound in a week, you must cut down or burn 3,500 calories per week or 500 calories per day. You would have to walk approximately 35 miles to burn one pound of fat. It would take about five hours of walking to get rid of one piece of pie—a half hour of bicycling to burn up one coke—an hour of steady dancing to burn up one piece of cake! But do not be discouraged; it is not necessary to do it in a day. If you take a daily half-hour walk, you could lose 10 pounds in a year. A half hour of tennis or badminton daily could result in a loss of 16 pounds in a year. *Exercise does burn calories* plus helping to maintain muscle strength and endurance and prevent flabbiness as weight is lost. Table XIX is an energy expenditure chart which may be helpful in determining the number of calories burned in some of your every day activities or sports. Table XX will allow you to estimate the number of calories you burn if you jog 1½ miles (see fitness tests in chapter 1).

It should be obvious that the heavier the person, the more calories burned. If you use the table to estimate your caloric expenditure, remember that the calculations are based on an hour's activity. If you wish to calculate expenditure per minute, multiply your weight times the number of calories per hour and then divide by 60. If you then exercise for only 20 minutes, multiply the caloric expenditure per minute by 20.

Another and perhaps more important reason for exercising is to avoid loss of muscle tissue during weight loss. Studies show that if you diet and do not exercise, you will lose not only fat tissue, but also large amounts of lean body mass. This loss of muscle (body protein) cannot be prevented by increasing protein in the diet. When one loses weight by exercise alone or by a combination of diet and exercise, the weight loss is mostly if not all fat and there may even be an increase in lean body mass, depending upon the type and intensity of exercise.

This is illustrated in a study[7] in which three groups of adult women had a 500 calorie per day deficit, either by cutting calorie intake, or increasing activity or both.(See Table XVIII). The three groups lost about the same amount of weight; however, there was a difference in the body composition. The two exercise groups lost more fat than did the Diet Group as well as increasing their lean body tissue. The Diet Group lost both fat and *muscle*. The change in body composition exhibited by these women supports our contention that the most satisfactory method of weight control is a combination of diet and exercise. As one doctor put it, "If 'homo laborans' becomes 'homo sedentarius' rather than 'homo sportius,' obesity will be an automatic consequence for many of our citizens.

Muscle tissue uses more calories than fat tissue. A lean person burns more calories than a fat person, and so finds it easier to stay slim. Calisthenics and weight training exercises which increase strength (and muscle mass) play as important a role in a "flab" control program as the higher energy burning aerobic exercises.

TABLE XVIII
Pounds of Tissue Lost With Diet and Exercise

	Lost Body Weight	Lost Body Fat	Lost or Gained Lean Body Tissue
Diet Group	−11.7	− 9.3	−2.4
Exercise Group	−10.6	−12.6	+2.0
Exercise-Diet Group	−12.0	−13.0	+1.0

One other aspect of exercise in weight and fat control is that *the increase in metabolism caused by the exercise may persist for hours after the activity has ceased, and thus continue to burn fat above that which was predicted.* For example, if you jog a mile, you might burn 125 calories, but you may actually burn an additional 25 or so calories in the hour following the run due to increased metabolism.

TABLE XIX
Approximate Number of Calories Used Per Pound of Body Weight*

Activities	Cal/hr./lb.	Activities	Cal/hr./lb.
Daily Activities		**Sports, Recreation, Dance, Exercise**	
Carpentry or farm chores	1.55	Calisthenics	2.00
Class Work, lecture	0.67	Canadian Air Force	
Cleaning Windows	1.65	5BX & XBX Chart I	3.31
Conversing	0.73	5BX & XBX Chart II	4.16
Chopping Wood	2.92	5BX & XBX Charts III & IV	5.86
Driving	1.20	XBX Charts V & VI	6.64
Dressing/Showering	1.27	Dancing	
Eating	0.56	(Aerobic)	
Floor (mopping/sweeping)	1.83	light	1.87
Gardening	1.42	moderate	3.00
Gardening & Weeding	2.35	vigorous	4.40
Hoeing, Raking, Planting	1.88	(Modern)	
House Painting/Metal Work	1.40	moderate	1.67
Housework	1.62	vigorous	2.27
Kneeling	0.47	(Fox Trot)	1.78
Laying Brick	1.36	(Rhumba)	2.77
Making Bed	1.57	(Square)	2.74
Mowing Grass (power mower)	1.62	(Waltz)	2.05
(push mower)	1.78	Hill Climbing	3.90
Office Work	1.20	Motorcycling	1.45
Pick & Shovel Work	2.68	Mountain Climbing	4.02
Repairing Car (mechanic)	1.67	Walking	
Resting in Bed	0.48	2 mph	1.40
Sawing Wood	3.12	110–120 paces/min.	2.07
Shining Shoes	1.18	4½ mph	2.65
Shoveling Snow	3.11	Stair, up and back down	
Sleeping	0.46	1 step @ 25 trips/min.	2.73
Standing (no activity)	0.57	1 step @ 30 trips/min.	2.93
(light activity)	0.98	1 step @ 35 trips/min.	3.33
Watching T.V.	0.47	3 steps @ 12 trips/min.	3.19
Working in Yard	1.41	5 steps @ 10 trips/min.	4.00
Writing	0.73	7 steps @ 9 trips/min.	4.80

*Adapted from Executive Fitness Newsletter, © 1975, 33 E. Minor Street, Emmaus, PA 18049.

Table XIX—*Continued*

Sports Activities	Cal/hr./lb.	Sports Activities	Cal/hr./lb.
Archery	2.05	Sailing (calm water)	1.20
Badminton (mod.)	2.27	Skating (moderate)	2.27
(vigorous)	3.90	(vigorous)	4.10
Baseball (infield/outfield)	1.88	Skiing (downhill)	3.87
(pitching)	2.33	(level 5 mph)	4.68
Basketball (moderate)	2.82	Soccer	3.58
(vigorous)	3.96	Squash	4.15
(half court)	1.67	Swim (backstroke)	
Bicycling on level, 5.5 mph	2.00	20 yds./min.	1.55
13.0 mph	4.30	25 yds./min.	1.93
Bowling, non-stop	2.67	30 yds./min.	2.12
Canoeing, 4 mph	2.82	35 yds./min.	2.74
Fencing (moderate)	2.00	40 yds./min.	3.34
(vigorous)	4.10	(breaststroke)	
Football	3.32	20 yds./min.	1.93
Golf (twosome)	1.16	30 yds./min.	2.89
(foursome)	1.62	40 yds./min.	3.85
Handball (vigorous)	3.90	(butterfly)	4.68
Ping Pong	3.77	(Crawl)	
Rope Jumping 110 jumps/min.	3.86	20 yds./min.	1.93
120 jumps/min.	3.73	45 yds./min.	3.48
130 jumps/min.	3.46	50 yds./min.	4.25
Rowing (pleasure)	2.00	(sidestroke)	3.34
Rowing Machine or sculling		Tennis (moderate)	2.77
20 strokes/min.	5.46	(vigorous)	3.90
Running (level) 5.5 mph	4.30	Volleyball	2.33
7 mph	5.59	Water Skiing	3.12
9 mph	6.21	Weight Training	3.13
12 mph	7.87	Wrestling/Judo/Karate	5.13
(in place) 140 cts./min.	9.76		

SUGGESTIONS FOR REDUCING

1. Consult your physician if you need to lose more than a few pounds. Weight reduction can actually be harmful.
2. Reduce caloric intake, but if you are not under a physician's supervision, do not reduce it below 1,000–1,200 calories. It is almost impossible to get an adequate supply of nutrients below this minimum. Do not waste your money on over-the-counter "diet pills."
3. Lose no more than one or two pounds per week unless you are under close medical supervision. After all, one pound a week is 52 pounds a year.

TABLE XX
The Caloric Cost of Running 1½ Miles (2.4 km)*

Weight (lbs.)	Calories/minute								
	8	9	10	11	12	13	14	15	16
120	125	124	121	120	119	117	116	114	112
130	135	133	132	130	128	126	125	123	121
140	145	143	141	139	138	136	134	132	130
150	155	153	151	149	147	145	143	141	139
160	165	163	161	159	156	154	152	150	148
170	175	173	170	168	166	164	161	159	157
180	185	182	180	178	175	173	171	168	166
190	195	192	190	187	185	182	180	177	175
200	205	202	199	197	194	192	189	186	184
210	215	212	209	206	204	201	198	195	193
220	225	222	219	216	213	210	207	204	202

*Adapted from Harger, B. S. Miller, J. B. and Thomas, J. C., "The Caloric Cost of Running: Its Impact on Weight Reduction," *Journal of the American Medical Association,* 228:4, 1974.

4. Combine your new eating habits with new exercise habits in a regimen you can live with a lifetime. It must be practical and fit your likes and dislikes.

5. Do not expect a steady loss of weight; because the body temporarily adjusts the metabolism to try to maintain weight, and because there will be periods of temporary water retention, you may appear to gain or stop losing when you know that you should be losing. This is a most difficult period, but "Hang in there, baby!"; eventually you will see the rewards.

6. Weigh only once a week (same time of day, same scales, same clothing). Weight may fluctuate as much as five pounds during the day under normal conditions and these temporary changes can be deceptive and discouraging. Graph your weight change in half pound increments until you reach your goal. (see Charts VI A and VI B in the Appendix.)

7. Diet and exercise with a friend or group who can reinforce you, share your victories and defeats, and help keep you working toward your goal.

8. Eat a balanced diet; cut down on (but do not eliminate) sugar, salt, fats, oils, and alcohol. One doughnut less per day means a loss of two pounds per month; substituting a baked potato for fried potatoes once a week can eliminate four pounds a year; substituting a glass of skim milk for a glass of whole milk makes a difference of eight pounds per year. (see Table XXI) Choose "*nutritionally dense*" food (low in calories-high in vitamins and minerals).

9. Avoid fad diets (see chapter 8 on Quackery and Fallacies); there is no food or drug which will take off pounds. It's a million-dollar racket, so don't believe the ads. Low-calorie, liquid-formula diets, containing all essential nutrients, are not practical for long periods except under close medical supervision; however, they may be effective when used at the beginning of a diet regimen or as a replacement for an occasional meal.

10. If you feel hungry on a three-meal diet reduce the size of the meal and add snacks for a fourth meal (but allow for the calories). Some studies show five small meals per day is better for reducing than three meals per day.

11. Watch it! Research shows obese people overeat in the evenings.

12. Eat breakfast to maintain your efficiency and help control your appetite at lunch. One-fourth of your daily caloric intake should be consumed at breakfast.

13. Eat many filling, low-calorie vegetables and complex carbohydrates; keep animal protein and fat low but the latter should not be less than 20% of your calories.

14. Do not use the "rhythm method of girth control"—gaining and losing repeatedly may be more harmful than maintaining a steady over-weight condition.

15. Record everything you eat, including the amount of the serving and the number of calories (see Charts IX and X in the Appendix). Eventually you will become "calorie wise" and learn to judge portions and calories. Refer to Tables XXI, XXII, in this chapter for ways to save calories. Refer to Table XXIII for a calorie counting guide.

SUGGESTIONS FOR GAINING

1. See your physician—you may need vitamin supplements or have other health problems needing attention.

2. Slow down—quit racing your engine; cut out the hurry by starting earlier. Plan ahead so you do not waste energy through inefficiency.

3. Get more rest and sleep; practice a conscious relaxation technique especially before meals (see Chapter 9).

4. Eat slowly and eat more; do not fill up on the bulky high cellulose foods.

5. Have a well-balanced diet of "nutritionally dense" foods—but high in calories as well as nutrients. Refer to Tables XXI and XXII for ways to increase calories. Refer to Table XXIII for help in finding high calorie foods.

6. Eat a hearty breakfast, and eat between meals if it does not dull your appetite. Five small meals a day might be more effective than three large meals.
7. Drink less fluid at meals and save room for the food.
8. Substitute milk for water when you are thirsty.
9. Do exercise for strength to increase the bulk of your muscles and perform rhythmical relaxation exercises.

HOW TO SUBSTITUTE FOODS

The overweight person can save an enormous number of calories which will never be missed, and the underweight person can increase caloric intake without being gluttonous, by substituting food of equal nutritional value and taste and quality, but with a caloric value to fit their needs. Whether you are on a weight-gaining or weight-losing diet or just trying to maintain your weight, it pays to become calorie wise. In the sample meals (Table XXI), the two extremes are compared to illustrate how the clever dieter can substitute foods.

TABLE XXI
Sample Meals*

Breakfast

High Cal	Calories	Low Cal	Calories
4 oz. orange juice	50	4 oz. orange juice	50
1 scrambled egg	120	1 boiled egg	78
2 slices bacon	100	1 slice bacon	50
2 slices white bread	126	2 slices gluten bread	70
2 pats butter	100	2 pats low cal margarine	34
2 cups coffee with 2 lumps		2 cups coffee with no-cal	
sugar and 2 tbsp. cream	220	sweetener and non-dairy cream	22
Total Calories	716	Total Calories	304

Lunch

Hamburger	350	Hamburger	350
1 slice apple pie	338	Low calorie pudding	123
1 glass (8 oz.) whole milk	165	1 glass (8 oz.) skim milk	80
Total Calories	853	Total Calories	553

*Used by permission of Pennwalt Prescription Products, *Are You Serious About Losing Weight,* Seventh Edition, 1973.

Table XXI—*Continued*

Dinner			
High Cal	**Calories**	**Low Cal**	**Calories**
½ glass (4 oz.) tomato juice	25	Consomme, 1 cup	10
6 oz. meat loaf with 4 tbsp. gravy	680	6 oz. club steak, broiled, lean	320
(41 calories per tbsp.)	164		
½ cup mashed potatoes	123	1 medium potato, baked	100
½ cup green peas	72	12 spears asparagus	40
2 slices French bread	160		
with 2 pats butter	100	2 pats low calorie margarine	34
Tossed salad	20	Hearts of lettuce	20
w/1½ tbsp. Roquefort		with low calorie salad	
Cheese dressing (100		dressing	15
calories per tbsp.)	150		
Iced plain layer cake	290	1 cup low calorie whipped	
		dessert	123
1 cup coffee with sugar		1 cup coffee with no-cal	
(2 lumps) and cream		sweetener and non-dairy	
(2 tbsp.)	110	cream	11
Total Calories	1,894	Total Calories	673

Snacks			
1 bottle cola beverage	105	Low calorie cola	2
1 custard (4 oz. cup)	205	2 low calorie cookies	50
1 cup coffee with sugar		1 cup coffee with no-cal	
(2 lumps) and cream		sweetener and non-dairy	
(2 tbsp.)	110	cream	11
1 small Danish pastry	140	2 low calorie cookies	50
Total Calories	560	Total Calories	113

Total Calories for day	4,023	Total Calories for day	1,643
		A saving of 2,380 calories	

Whether you are trying to gain or lose, Table XXII can be helpful. It provides a list of foods in the left hand column which are relatively high in calories and in the right hand column, there is an alternate but comparable food which is lower in calories. The foods are grouped into categories for easier reference. If you are trying to lose weight/fat, substitute the foods in the "Low Cal" column for those in the "High Cal" column. If you are trying to increase your weight, then of course you should choose the "High Cal" column. The number of calories difference between the two choices is given in the column labeled "Difference."

TABLE XXII
List of Foods Which Can Be Substituted for More or Less Calories*

High Cal	Calories	Low Cal	Calories	Difference
		Beverages		
Milk (whole) 8 oz.	165	Milk (buttermilk or skim) 8 oz.	80	85
Prune juice, 8 oz.	170	Tomato Juice, 8 oz.	50	120
Soft drinks, 8 oz.	105	Diet soft drinks, 8 oz.	1	104
Coffee, cream, 2 tsp. sugar	110	Coffee (black with artificial sweetener)	0	110
Cocoa (all milk), 8 oz.	235	Cocoa (milk & water), 8 oz.	140	95
Chocolate malt, 8 oz.	500	Lemonade (sweetened), 8 oz.	100	400
Beer, 12 oz.	175	Lite Beer	100	75
		Breakfast Foods		
Rice Flakes, 1 cup	110	Puffed Rice, 1 cup	50	60
Eggs (scrambled), 2	220	Eggs (boiled/poached) 2	160	60
		Butter and Cheese		
Butter on toast	170	Apple butter on toast	90	80
Cheese (Blue, Cheddar, Cream, Swiss), 1 oz.	105	Cheese (cottage, uncreamed), 1 oz.	25	80
		Desserts		
Angel food cake, 2" piece	110	Cantaloupe melon, ½	40	70
Cheese cake, 2" piece	200	Watermelon, ½" slice (10" diam.)	60	140
Chocolate cake with icing, 2" piece	425	Sponge cake, 2" piece	120	305
Fruit cake, 2" piece	115	Grapes, 1 cup	65	50
Pound cake, 1 oz. piece	140	Plums, 2	50	90
Cupcake, white icing, 1	230	Plain cupcake, 1	115	115
Cookies, assorted (3" diam.), 1	120	Vanilla wafer (dietetic), 1	25	95
Ice cream, 4 oz.	150	Yogurt (flavored), 4 oz.	60	90
		Pies		
Apple, 1 piece (1/7 of a 9" pie)	345	Tangerine (fresh), 1	40	305
Blueberry, 1 piece	290	Blueberries (frozen, unsweetened), ½ cup	45	245
Cherry, 1 piece	355	Cherries (whole), ½ cup	40	315
Custard, 1 piece	280	Banana, small, 1	85	195

*Used by permission of Pennwalt Prescription Products, *Are You Serious About Losing Weight,* Seventh Edition, 1973.

Table XXII—*Continued*

High Cal	Calories	Low Cal	Calories	Difference
Lemon meringue, 1 piece	305	Lemon flavored gelatin, ½ cup	70	235
Peach, 1 piece	280	Peach, (whole), 1	35	245
Rhubarb, 1 piece	265	Grapefruit, ½	55	210
Pudding (flavored), ½ cup	140	Pudding (dietetic, non-fat milk), ½ cup	60	80

Fish and Fowl

High Cal	Calories	Low Cal	Calories	Difference
Tuna (canned), 3 oz.	165	Crabmeat (canned), 3 oz.	80	85
Oysters (fried), 6	400	Oysters (shell w/sauce) 6	100	300
Ocean perch (fried), 4 oz.	260	Bass, 4 oz.	105	155
Fish sticks, 5 sticks or 4 oz.	200	Swordfish (broiled), 3 oz.	140	60
Lobster meat, 4 oz. with 2 tbsp. butter	300	Lobster meat, 4 oz. with lemon	95	205
Duck (roasted), 3 oz.	310	Chicken (roasted), 3 oz.	160	150

Meats

High Cal	Calories	Low Cal	Calories	Difference
Loin roast, 3 oz.	290	Pot roast (round), 3 oz.	160	130
Rump roast, 3 oz.	290	Rib roast, 3 oz.	200	90
Swiss steak, 3½ oz.	300	Liver (fried), 2½ oz.	210	90
Hamburger (av. fat, broiled), 3 oz.	240	Hamburger (lean, broiled), 3 oz.	145	95
Porterhouse steak, 3 oz.	250	Club steak, 3 oz.	160	90
Rib lamb chop (med.), 3 oz.	300	Veal chop (med.), 3 oz.	160	140
Pork chop (med.), 3 oz.	340	Veal chop (med.), 3 oz.	185	155
Pork roast, 3 oz.	310	Veal roast, 3 oz.	230	80
Pork sausage, 3 oz.	405	Ham (boiled, lean), 3 oz.	200	205

Potatoes

High Cal	Calories	Low Cal	Calories	Difference
Fried, 1 cup	480	Baked (2½" diam.)	100	380
Mashed, 1 cup	245	Boiled (2½" diam.)	100	140

Salads

High Cal	Calories	Low Cal	Calories	Difference
Chef salad with oil dressing, 1 tbsp.	180	Chef salad with dietetic dressing, 1 tbsp.	40	120
Chef salad with mayonnaise, 1 tbsp.	125	Chef salad with dietetic dressing, 1 tbsp.	40	85
Chef salad with Roquefort, Blue, Russian, French dressing, 1 tbsp.	105	Chef salad with dietetic dressing, 1 tbsp.	40	65

Table XXII—*Continued*

High Cal	Calories	Low Cal	Calories	Difference
		Sandwiches		
Club	375	Bacon and tomato (open)	200	175
Peanut butter and jelly	275	Egg salad (open)	165	110
Turkey with gravy, 3 tbsp.	520	Hamburger, lean, (open) 3 oz.	200	320
		Snacks		
Fudge, 1 oz.	115	Vanilla wafers (dietetic), 2	50	65
Peanuts (salted), 1 oz.	170	Apple, 1	100	70
Peanuts (roasted), 1 cup shelled	1,375	Grapes, 1 cup	65	1,305
Potato chips, 10 med.	115	Pretzels, 10 small sticks	35	80
Chocolate, 1 oz. bar	145	Toasted marshmallows, 3	75	70
		Soups		
Creamed, 1 cup	210	Chicken noodle, 1 cup	110	100
Bean, 1 cup	190	Beef noodle, 1 cup	110	80
Minestrone, 1 cup	105	Beef bouillon, 1 cup	10	95
		Vegetables		
Baked beans, 1 cup	320	Green beans, 1 cup	30	290
Lima beans, 1 cup	160	Asparagus, 1 cup	30	130
Corn (canned), 1 cup	185	Cauliflower, 1 cup	30	155
Peas (canned), 1 cup	145	Peas (fresh), 1 cup	115	30
Winter squash, 1 cup	75	Summer squash, 1 cup	30	45
Succotash, 1 cup	260	Spinach, 1 cup	40	200

Most experts agree that the successful dieter must learn about the caloric value of food. Even though you choose to follow a diet prescribed by someone who has already counted the calories for you, sooner or later you will need to modify your eating patterns on a permanent basis if you wish to maintain your weight/fat at a constant desirable level. Therefore it is inevitable that you refer to a table such as The Calorie Guide to Common Foods, Table XXIII. (You will need this Table when you complete Charts IX and X in the Appendix).

TABLE XXIII
Calorie Guide to Common Foods

Beverages		Dairy Products	
Coffee (black)	3	Butter, 1 pat (1½ tsp.)	50
Coke (12 oz.)	137	Cheese, cheddar (1 oz.)	113
Hot chocolate, milk (1 cup)	247	Cheese, cottage (1 cup)	270
Lemonade (1 cup)	100	Cheese, cream (1 oz.)	106
Limeade, diluted to serve (1 cup)	110	Cheese, Parmesan (1 tbsp.)	29
Soda, fruit flavored (12 oz.)	161	Cheese, Swiss natural (1 oz.)	105
Tea (clear)	3	Cream, sour (1 tbsp.)	31
Breads and Cereals		Dairy Queen cone (med.)	335
Bagel (1 half)	76	Frozen custard (1 cup)	375
Biscuit (2″ × 2″)	135	Frozen yogurt, vanilla (1 cup)	180
Bread, Pita (1 oz.)	80	Ice cream, plain (prem.) (1 cup)	350
Bread, raisin (½″ thick)	65	Ice cream soda, choc. (large glass)	455
Bread, rye	55	Ice milk (1 cup)	184
Bread, white enriched (½″ thick)	64	Ices (1 cup)	177
Bread, whole wheat (½″ thick)	55	Milk, chocolate (1 cup)	185
Bun (hamburger)	120	Milk, half-and-half (1 tbsp.)	20
Cereals, cooked (½ cup)	80	Milk, malted (1 cup)	281
Corn flakes (1 cup)	96	Milkshake (White Castle)	213
Corn grits (1 cup)	125	Milk, skim (1 cup)	88
Corn muffin (2½″ diam.)	103	Milk, skim dry (1 tbsp.)	28
Crackers, graham (1 med.)	28	Milk, whole (1 cup)	166
Crackers, soda (1 plain)	24	Sherbert (1 cup)	270
English muffin (1 half)	74	Whipped topping (1 tbsp.)	14
Macaroni, with cheese (1 cup)	464	Yogurt (1 cup)	150
Muffin, plain	135	**Desserts and Sweets**	
Noodles (1 cup)	200	Banana split (Dairy Queen)	547
Oatmeal (1 cup)	150	Cake, angel (2″ wedge)	108
Pancakes (1–4″ diam.)	59	Cake, chocolate (2″ × 3″ × 1″)	150
Pizza (1 section)	180	Cake, plain (3″ × 2½″)	180
Popped corn (1 cup)	54	Chocolate, bar	200–300
Potato chips (10 med.)	108	Chocolate, bitter (1 oz.)	142
Pretzels (5 small sticks)	18	Chocolate, sweet (1 oz.)	133
Rice (1 cup)	225	Chocolate, syrup (1 tbsp.)	42
Roll, plain (1 med.)	118	Cinnamon roll (White Castle)	305
Roll, sweet (1 med.)	178	Cocoa (1 tbsp.)	21
Shredded wheat (1 med. biscuit)	79	Cookies, plain (1 med.)	75
Spaghetti, plain cooked (1 cup)	218	Custard, baked (1 cup)	283
Tortilla (1 corn)	70	Doughnut (1 large)	250
Waffle (4½″ × 5″)	216		

Note: For a complete listing of foods, the reader is referred to: *Nutritive Value of Foods,* U.S. Department of Agriculture, Washington, D.C., Home and Gardens Bulletin, No. 72. (Available in most libraries, university bookstores, and Home Economics departments).

Table XXIII—*Continued*

Gelatin, dessert (1 cup)	155	**Meat, Fish, Eggs**	
Gelatin, with fruit (1 cup)	170	Bacon, drained (2 slices)	97
Gingerbread (2″ × 2″ × 2″)	180	Bacon, Canadian (1 oz.)	62
Jams, jellies (1 tbsp.)	55	Beef, hamburger chuck (3 oz.)	316
Pie, apple (1/7 of 9″ pie)	345	Beef, pot pie	560
Pie, apple (McDonalds)	265	Beef steak, sirloin or T-bone (3 oz.)	257
Pie, cherry (1/7 of 9″ pie)	355	Beef and vegetable stew (1 cup)	185
Pie, chocolate (1/7 of 9″ pie)	360	Chicken, fried breast (8 oz.)	210
Pie, coconut (1/7 of 9″ pie)	266	Chicken, fried (1 leg and thigh)	305
Pie, lemon meringue (1/7 of 9″ pie)	302	Chicken, fried (Colonel Sanders 3-piece special)	660
Sugar, granulated (1 tsp.)	27	Chicken, roasted breast (2 slices)	100
Syrup, table (1 tbsp.)	57	Chili, without beans (1 cup)	510
Fruit		Chili, with beans (1 cup)	335
Apple, fresh (med.)	76	Egg, boiled	77
Applesauce, unsweetened (1 cup)	184	Egg, fried	125
Avocado, raw (½ peeled)	279	Egg, scrambled	100
Banana, fresh (med.)	88	Fish and Chips (2 pcs. fish; 4 oz. chips Arthur Treacher's)	275
Cantaloupe, raw (½, 5″ diam.)	60	Fish, broiled (3″ × 3″ × ½″)	112
Cherries (10 sweet)	50	Fish stick	40
Cranberry sauce, unsweetened (1 tbsp.)	25	Frankfurter, boiled	124
Fruit cocktail, canned (1 cup)	170	Ham (4″ × 4″)	338
Grapefruit, fresh (½)	60	Lamb (3 oz. roast, lean)	158
Grapefruit, juice, raw (1 cup)	95	Liver (3″ × 3″)	150
Grape juice, bottled (½ cup)	80	Luncheon meat (2 oz.)	135
Grapes (20–25)	75	Pork chop, loin (3″ × 5″)	284
Nectarine (1 med.)	88	Salmon, canned (1 cup)	145
Olives, green (10)	72	Sausage, pork (4 oz.)	510
Olives, ripe (10)	105	Shrimp, canned (3 oz.)	108
Orange, fresh (med.)	60	Tuna, canned (½ cup)	185
Orange juice, frozen diluted (1 cup)	110	Veal, cutlet (3″ × 4″)	175
Peach, fresh (med.)	46	**Nuts and Seeds**	
Peach, canned in syrup (2 halves)	79	Cashews (1 cup)	770
Pear, fresh (med.)	95	Coconut (1 cup)	450
Pears, canned in syrup (2 halves)	79	Peanut butter (1 tbsp.)	92
Pineapple, crushed in syrup (1 cup)	204	Peanuts, roasted, no skin (1 cup)	805
Pineapple (½ cup fresh)	50	Pecans (1 cup)	752
Prune juice (1 cup)	170	Sunflower seeds, (1 tbsp.)	50
Raisins, dry (1 tbsp.)	26	**Sandwiches and Mexican Fast Food**	
Strawberries, fresh (1 cup)	54	(2 slices of bread—plain)	
Strawberries, frozen (3 oz.)	90	Bologna	214
Tangerine (2½″ diam.)	40	Burrito (Taco Bell)	319
Watermelon, wedge (4″ × 8″)	120		

Table XXIII—*Continued*

Cheeseburger (small McDonald)	300	**Vegetables**	
Cheeseburger (Wendy's Triple)	1,430	Alfalfa sprouts (½ cup)	19
Chicken salad	185	Asparagus (6 spears)	22
Egg salad	240	Bean sprouts (1 cup)	37
Egg McMuffin (McDonald's)	312	Beans, Frijoles (Taco Bell)	178
Fish Filet (McDonald's)	400	Beans, green (1 cup)	27
Fish (Burger King "Whaler")	744	Beans, lima (1 cup)	152
Ham	360	Beans, navy (1 cup)	642
Ham and cheese	360	Beans, pork and molasses (1 cup)	325
Ham and cheese (Arby's)	458	Broccoli, fresh cooked (1 cup)	60
Hamburger (small McDonald's)	260	Cabbage, cooked (1 cup)	40
Hamburger (Burger King Whopper)	600	Cauliflower (1 cup)	25
Hamburger (Big Mac)	550	Carrot, raw (med.)	21
Hamburger (McDonald's Quarter Pounder)	420	Carrots, canned (1 cup)	44
		Celery, diced raw (1 cup)	20
Hamburger (Burger King)	252	Coleslaw (1 cup)	102
Peanut butter	250	Corn, sweet, canned (1 cup)	140
Roast Beef (Arby's Regular)	425	Corn, sweet (med. ear)	84
Roast Beef (Arby's Super)	705	Cucumber, raw (6 slices)	6
Sauces, Fats, Oils		Lettuce (2 large leaves)	7
Catsup, tomato (1 tbsp.)	17	Mushrooms, canned (1 cup)	28
Chili sauce (1 tbsp.)	17	Onions, french fried (10 rings)	75
French dressing (1 tbsp.)	59	Onions, raw (med.)	25
Margarine (1 pat)	50	Peas, field (½ cup)	90
Mayonnaise (1 tbsp.)	92	Peas, green (1 cup)	145
Mayonnaise-type (1 tbsp.)	65	Pickles, dill (med.)	15
Taco (Taco Bell)	159	Pickles, sweet (med.)	22
Tostado (Taco Bell)	188	Potato, baked (med.)	97
Turkey (Arby's without dressing)	337	Potato, french fried (8 sticks)	155
Vegetable, sunflower, safflower oils (1 tbsp.)	120	Potato, mashed (1 cup)	185
		Radish, raw (small)	1
Soup, Ready to Serve		Sauerkraut, drained (1 cup)	32
Bean (1 cup)	190	Spinach, fresh, cooked (1 cup)	46
Beef noodle	100	Squash, summer (1 cup)	30
Cream	200	Sweet pepper (med.)	15
Tomato	90	Sweet potato, candied (small)	314
Vegetable	80	Tomato, cooked (1 cup)	50
		Tomato, raw (med.)	30

REFERENCES

1. National Institutes of Health, *Health Implications of Obesity,* National Institutes of Health Consensus Development Conference Statement, U.S. Department of Health and Human Services, Public Health Service, N.I.H., Bethesda, Maryland, 5:9 (1985).
2. Burton, B. T., Foster, W. R., Hirsch, J. and Van Itallie, T. B., "Health Implications of Obesity: An NIH Consensus Development Conference," *International Journal of Obesity,* 9:(1985):155–170.
3. "Height-Weights Used as Dietary Guidelines," *Nutrition Week,* Feb. 21, 1985, pp. 5–6.
4. Burton, B. T. and Foster, W. R., "Health Implications of Obesity: An NIH Consensus Development Conference," *Journal of the American Dietetic Association,* 85:9 (Sept. 1985):1117–1121.
5. U.S. Department of Agriculture, *Dietary Guidelines for Americans,* 2nd Ed., Home & Garden Bulletin No. 332, Washington, D.C., 1985.
6. Connor, S. L. and Connor, W. E., *The New American Diet,* New York, Simon and Schuster, 1986, p. 166.
7. Zuti, M. B., "Effects of Diet and Exercise on Body Composition of Adult Women During Weight Reduction," doctoral dissertation, Kent State University, 1972, as reported in *Physical Fitness Research Digest,* President's Council on Physical Fitness, Washington, D.C., 5:2 (April, 1975).
8. Division of Chronic Diseases, Heart Disease Control Program, *Obesity and Health,* Washington, D.C.: Public Health Service, U.S. Department of Health, Education and Welfare, 43.

RESOURCES

1. American Anorexia Nervosa Assn., Inc.
   133 Cedar Lane
   Teaneck, New Jersey 07666
   Phone: 201-836-1800
2. National Anorexic Aid Society, Inc.
   P.O. Box 29461
   Columbus, Ohio 43229
   Phone: 614-846-6810
3. The National Association of Anorexia Nervosa and Associated Disorders
   Box 271
   Highland Park, Illinois 60035
   Phone 312-831-3438

Quackery and Fallacies

7

look up def of nutrition of dictionary of cellulite

PRETEST

1. What is a fad diet?
2. Should everyone take vitamin and mineral supplements "just in case"?
3. Can you massage away fat?
4. Can you melt off fat in a sauna bath?
5. Is cellulite a special kind of fat that requires a special kind of reducing treatment?
6. Is figure wrapping a safe and effective reducing technique?
7. How qualified are the instructors in most health clubs and reducing salons to give advice on health, fitness, and reducing?
8. Can you take off fat from your hips by doing hip exercises?

Quacks and hucksters are bilking the public of millions of dollars each year on gadgets, so-called health foods, diets, and pills which are useless and sometimes even harmful. Radio, television, newspapers, and books frequently carry false or misleading advertisements and incorrect information about exercise and weight control. Surveys show that a large percentage of people believe that if something is "in print" or is said "on the air," then it must be true. Unfortunately, this is not the case because our laws and means of enforcing them are inadequate to prevent most of the hoaxes perpetrated on the consumer. The only real protection is the educated consumer.

FAD DIETS

There are hundreds of fad diets, usually designed to sell books or special ingredients in the diet. Typically these diets manipulate protein, fat, and carbohydrates so that one or two components are markedly increased while the other(s) is/are drastically decreased or eliminated. The dangers in such unbalanced diets include:

No or Low Fat Diet—may lead to hunger, irritability, dry skin and scalp, stiff joints, constipation, poor concentration, and general unhealthiness.

High Fat Diet (usually combined with high protein and low carbohydrate)—may cause diarrhea, loss of nutrients and electrolytes, and high cholesterol levels (this may cause heart disease).

No or Low Carbohydrate (usually combined with high protein and high fat)—may cause excessive retention of uric acid, gout, kidney problems, complications for the diabetic or pregnant woman, hypoglycemia, dizziness, weakness, dehydration, nausea, or irritability.

No or Low Protein—may result in weakness and loss of muscle and organ tissues; it is dangerous to fall below 70 grams.

No juggling of nutrients is effective in making you lose weight or gain weight unless you also restrict calorie intake. Calories do count. Whether you count them or follow a pre-counted diet, it is the number of calories rather than the source of the calories which ultimately determines weight loss/gain.

DIET FOODS AND SUPPLEMENTS

All foods contain calories. There is **no** such thing as a reducing food, negative calorie food, or food with special ability to burn off fat. Grapefruit is **not** a yellow spark-plug. Protein supplements will **not** make you lose weight. A liquid protein diet is **not** a safe way to reduce as it may cause an irregular heart beat which can be fatal. Safflower oil does **not** loosen long-stored fat. Vinegar, vitamin B_6, and lecithin have **no** beneficial properties in a weight or fat loss program. Diet beer, diet chocolate pudding, diet bars, etc., contain calories, and eaten in enough quantity can make you gain. Water has **no** calories and is **not** a food, but many people on a water diet think that the eight glasses of water per day make the diet successful. Sunflower seed oil is **no** lower in calories or cholesterol than are other vegetable oils. Everyone does **not** need to take vitamin and mineral supplements. It is possible to "O.D." on vitamins. Prolonged overdosing of vitamin C, for example, can cause kidney stones, diarrhea, and heart burn. Sudden withdrawal can cause scurvy-like symptoms. Other vitamins and supplements similarly cause toxicity when abused.

Another example of toxicity is seen in the multiple sclerosis type symptoms produced in patients taking vitamin B_6 in megadoses (as treatment for premenstrual syndrome). It is **not** true that vitamin C prevents colds. At least 16 double blind studies over the past 10 years have disproven this myth. Neither does vitamin C prolong the lives of cancer patients. Contrary to earlier reports, vitamin E does **not** help rid women of lumps in the breast. There is **no** scientific evidence that bee pollen has any beneficial effects on athletic performance, weight control, or health, as its manufacturers claim.

DRUGS FOR REDUCING

Prescription Drugs

In the 1950s–60s, obesity clinics freely prescribed a potent combination of drugs known as "Rainbow Pills" which included amphetamines, barbiturates, thyroid, digitalis, diuretics, laxatives, antispasmodies, and hypotensive agents. These resulted in so many cases of deafness, blindness, paralysis, and even death that the government has drastically limited the writing of such prescriptions. Besides being dangerous in combinations, many of them are addictive, and all merely serve as crutches, while failing to change the eating patterns of the patients.

Over-the-Counter Drugs

There are probably a thousand or more non-prescription reducing drugs available, all of which are ineffective; as quickly as the Food and Drug Administration (FDA) removes them from the market, they reappear under a new name. There are bulk producers (such as glucomanan) which it is claimed will fill the stomach and reduce hunger pains, but which actually work only in the intestines and have **no** effect on appetite. There are appetite depressants, such as those containing phenylpropanolamine (p.p.a. or propradine). In spite of the fact that the FDA approved this drug, studies show it to be ineffective in the recommended doses and if larger doses are taken, especially by those with heart disease, thyroid problems, high blood pressure, and diabetes, it may be dangerous. Starch blockers are believed to be ineffective as well as unsafe.

LOTIONS, CREAMS, DIET CANDY, DIET CHEWING GUM, AND DIET CIGARETTES

These are equally ineffective in a weight or girth control program. There is **nothing** known to modern science which is safe and effective for you to rub on, drink, chew, or smoke to lose weight. Accustaple (staples in the ears) has **not** been proven effective. Injections of human chorionic gonadotropin (HCG) lack scientific evidence of effectiveness. Generally, one may assume that anyone who claims to have a quick and easy cure is a quack.

GADGETS AND GIMMICKS

Passive Exercise Machines

Passive exercise, in which a machine or another person moves your body with little or no effort on your part, is useless for weight or girth reduction. Examples of some of these ineffective devices include:

Rollers—whether hand-held or motor driven, these wooden or metal cylinders have **no** effect on weight, shape, or fat when rolled up and down on the body part.

Vibrating Belts, Tables, and Pillows—these gadgets which shake the person or body part do **not** "break-up fatty deposits," improve posture, or take off inches.

Motor Driven Bicycles and Rowing Machines—these devices move the arms and legs of the rider who sits passively. They contribute **nothing** to the fitness or girth control of the normal person.

Massage—whether given by a mechanical device or by a masseur, this manipulation of the tissues is passive. It may have some therapeutic benefits but it does **not** aid in improving fitness or figure/physique.

Sauna, Steam, and Whirlpool Baths

Dry sauna, wet sauna, steam baths, whirlpool baths, hot tubs, and other forms of applying heat and water are claimed by their proponents to do everything from melting off pounds to curing bronchitis, improving complexion, and "ridding the body of toxins and poisons." One sauna manufacturer even claims his device cures cancer! The truth is, they do **none** of these things and poorly maintained hot tubs can help spread contagious skin bacteria and herpes virus. Some people enjoy the largely psychological effect of the baths and find them relaxing. Persons with chronic arthritis, sprains, bruises, and muscle soreness may find temporary relief induced by the heat; but the same beneficial effects can be obtained by sitting in a tub of hot water at home. The heat in the baths will cause the body to perspire and lose body fluids (dehydrate). Dehydration causes a temporary loss of weight until the water is replaced by normal eating and drinking. The baths do **not** melt off fat.

Sauna and steam baths can be dangerous for the elderly, or for bathers suffering from asthma, vascular problems, kidney dysfunction, metabolic disorders, diabetes, heart trouble, and high blood pressure, as well as those under the influence of hypnotics, narcotics, or tranquilizers. This is **not** a good way to get rid of a hangover. Prolonged exposure can result in severe dehydration, causing not only water loss but also a deprivation of mineral salts. This can lead to heat stroke and, eventually, to brain damage and death.

If you do use them, the maximum temperature of the sauna should be 190° F and the steam bath should not exceed 120° F. Beginners should limit their stay to a maximum of six minutes while experienced users should stay no longer than 15 minutes. After the bath, drink plenty of water to replace lost fluids; shower and shampoo to thoroughly remove residual salts, acids, metals, or chemicals and then moisturize your skin.

Non-Porous Garments

"Melts pounds away as you work or play," says the advertisement for non-porous garments such as sauna suits (jeans, shorts, belts, sleepwear, and girdles). These garments have been on the market for a number of years under a variety of trade names. They are made of material (such as rubber) which is non-porous and holds in body heat, causing perspiration and/or they fit tightly and may even be inflatable. The latter varieties of air belts and shorts are like plastic innertubes which serve as constricting bands as well as non-porous garments.

Perspiration causes dehydration and a temporary weight loss of body fluids (**not** a fat loss); weight is regained as soon as liquids are replaced. Constricting bands can squeeze the superficial fluids into deeper tissues of the body and cause a temporary indentation and decrease in girth just as a tight watch band leaves an indentation on the wrist. These bands do not squeeze out fat and have **no** value. They may even cause medical problems by interfering with blood flow in the veins from the lower extremities back to the heart.

Weighted Belts

Belts containing lead granules and weighing six to nine pounds have been advertised to be worn under clothing throughout the day for weight loss, waist slimming, and physical fitness. One study showed it would take a 200 pound man 45 days to burn enough calories to lose one pound. These belts not only have been found to be **ineffective,** but they were ordered off the market by the government because they resulted in injuries to the lower back and caused joint strain.

Muscle Stimulators

A variety of electronic "effortless exercise" devices have been on the market since the 1930s, which claim to "tone flabby muscles" and cause a girth reduction. These are muscle stimulators, similar to those used in hospital physical therapy departments, which send an electric current into the muscle, causing it to contract involuntarily. Some of these devices might actually be effective in producing a mild strengthening effect and preventing muscle atrophy, but are **not** as effective as voluntary muscle contractions used in exercises; furthermore, they could be very dangerous in the hands of the public. Government agencies have attempted to remove some of these machines from the market because they have been found to aggravate many medical conditions.

Bust Developers

Charlatans have offered a variety of gimmicks purported to enlarge the female breasts—lotions, hormone creams, suction pumps, water massage, electrical muscle stimulators, and exercise devices. The breasts, of course, are mammary glands composed largely of fatty tissue and suspended by ligaments. They are not muscles and **cannot** be exercised or stimulated to contract. The breast lies on top of the pectoralis major, a large muscle on the chest; when the pectoral muscle is strengthened it increases in mass (hypertrophy), and causes an increase in the chest girth; there is **no** way to increase the size of the breasts other than augmentation surgery (silicon transplants) or silicon injections. The latter are considered unsafe.

Cellulite

One fraud is the claim that eight out of ten women have a "fat-gone-wrong" called cellulite (pronounced sell-u-leet) that will not respond to diet and exercise. Presumably, it looks dimpled like orange peeling and needs special treatment. This **rip-off** is used to sell books and strange treatments such as a stream of hot air directed on a body part while an automated suction massage machine works on the fat. This is bunk! The word *cellulite* is not likely to be found in medical books; it refers to ordinary superficial adipose tissue—fat, which may or may not look like orange peel, but which will be lost only when there is a calorie deficit.

Figure Wrapping

Some reducing salons and mail order establishments claim you can lose from four to 12 inches in one treatment, with no diet and no exercise. The treatment consists of a hot shower, followed by being wrapped like a mummy in linen bandages dipped in a "magic solution," then an hour of waiting encased in a sauna suit in a cold room. The solutions vary, but are apt to be epsom salts (magnesium sulfate and aluminum sulfate), glycerin, and herbs and spices. There is a slight, temporary decrease in girth measurements due to the constricting pressure squeezing body fluids to deeper tissues and the hypertonic effect of the solution which tends to dehydrate the superficial tissues. The cold room may produce further body shrinkage from hypothermia, as the blood vessels constrict to conserve heat. These effects are **temporary** and will disappear in a few hours. The treatment is **dangerous,** has caused the death of at least one woman, and can be harmful to those with heart or circulatory problems, varicose veins, phlebitis, or kidney trouble.

Tanning Booths/Salons

The rapidly growing suntanning industry claims their equipment is safe because it reduces or eliminates Ultraviolet-B (UV-B) rays and increases UV-A rays which have less potential for burning. However, UV-A penetrates the skin more deeply and can produce wrinkled, leathery, prematurely aged skin. While UV-B has a well established risk factor for skin cancer, some studies show UV-A may increase the cancer-producing potential of UV-B. In addition, large doses of UV-A can harm the cornea and lens of the eye and either one of the rays may cause cataracts with repeated exposure. Both the Food and Drug Administration and the American Medical Association warn against using suntanning lamps.

Reducing Salons, Health Clubs, Spas

The Negative Side. The typical establishment is a highly commercial business more interested in making a profit than in the welfare of the client. Its personnel are not qualified and rarely have degrees or certificates in physical therapy, physical education, or corrective therapy. Most are hired for their nice appearance and are trained on the job in a few short weeks. They are not qualified to diagnose and prescribe for health, figure/physique, or fitness problems. Most establishments offer all the passive exercise gimmicks and baths, and some include figure wrapping and the prescription of fad diets. Most provide active exercise programs and weight lifting equipment, also, but they rarely give training for cardiovascular endurance. Many of the treatment claims are false or misleading, and some of their programs can be harmful. John Dietrich's 1983 survey substantiated what Lindsey found in 1971, that is, "99 percent of the clubs do not offer adequate exercise instruction and most of them apply high-pressure sales tactics to get you to sign up or risk losing a 'special discount.' "[1,2]

The Positive Side. There are some worthwhile clubs which emphasize exercise, rather than just socialization and relaxation. Some are full service fitness facilities with lap pools, aerobic classes, and aerobic equipment (treadmills, rowing machines, and exercise bikes) as well as weight resistance machines. A few clubs even offer an indoor track for joggers. Then there are specialty clubs such as the Nautilus equipment centers and body building gyms emphasizing free weights where the serious client can develop strength and endurance. There are some good commercial fitness centers with qualified personnel (with degrees in physical education, corrective therapy, physical therapy, or exercise physiology). Diet clubs such as Tops and Weight Watchers are also reputable, but you would need to provide your own exercise program if you joined one of these. Aerobic dance exercise classes are offered everywhere but you will not always find trained instructors. Health clubs do offer facilities and equipment and a pleasant place to meet and exercise with your friends (at a price), but as a general rule, it would be better to investigate programs offered by the local YMCA-YWCA, parks and recreation departments, university, and community colleges.

The moral is, you can save your money and exercise at home, but if you need the motivation provided by a group setting, select the club carefully, giving most of your attention to the qualification of the instructor.

CHOOSING A CLUB

If you choose to join a club, the following check list may help you make a wise choice. The answers to the first nine questions should be "no." Questions 10–14 should be answered "yes," if you want the best. You should recognize that some of these questions are more important than others and should be weighted in making your decision.

Health Club Evaluation Check List*

1. Do they advertise or promise "miraculous" results?
2. Do they use high pressure salesmanship?
3. Do they try to sell you a long term contract?
4. Is the contract non-cancellable?
5. Do they "push" diets and food supplements as a side line?
6. Do they pester you to bring in new members?
7. Do they limit the number of minutes you can use a piece of equipment?
8. Do they have passive equipment or offer "effortless" exercise?
9. Are the facilities over-crowded during the hours you would normally participate?
10. Do they have facilities and/or equipment for cardiovascular training? (a) lap pool (b) track (c) aerobic gym (d) bicycle ergometers (e) other
11. Do their hours fit your schedule?
12. Do the instructors have degrees in physical education, exercise physiology, physical therapy, kinesiotherapy, or kinesiology?
13. Do they have clean dressing rooms and showers?
14. Are the other clients the types of people you would enjoy socializing with?
15. Could you get the same benefits for less at your local Y, community college or recreation center?

FALLACIES AND MISCONCEPTIONS

There are a number of fallacies and misconceptions in the weight and fatness control and physical fitness areas. Some of these are included below along with brief statements regarding the true facts.

Fallacy 1: *Obesity is caused by gluttony.*

Chapter 6 briefly described some of the causes of obesity, including the summary statement that the overweight (fat) person consumes more calories than are burned. This is a correct concept, but it often is misinterpreted to mean that fat people are gluttons. Most overweight is of the "creeping" kind caused by a gradual slow-down in activity and metabolism as we get older, without an accompanying decrease in our caloric consumption. There are some gluttons among the obese, but there are many more who eat less than their non-fat counterparts. When they say, "But I hardly eat enough to keep a bird alive," for some, it may be true. Several studies of boys and girls have shown that the fat ones ate less than their normal weight peers, but were less active physically. Similar studies on adults and animals confirm that *inactivity contributes to much obesity.*

*Adapted from Corbin, C. and Lindsey, R., *Concepts in Physical Fitness,* 6th edition Dubuque, Iowa, Wm. C. Brown Publishers, 1988.

Fallacy 2: *Exercise increases the appetite and therefore should be avoided by a person trying to reduce.*

Both animal and human studies carried out by nutritionists refute this idea. The sedentary person who begins an exercise program will usually take in more food than is burned in activity and will gain weight. The normally active person will tend to increase food intake, but it will be balanced by the activity output so that no weight is gained. The person who exercises to exhaustion will tend to lose both appetite and weight.

Fallacy 3: *Exercising the spot where fat is deposited will make the fat come off of that spot.*

As previously mentioned, the location of fat deposits is controlled genetically and differs somewhat from person to person. If too much of it is deposited in a spot where we do not want it, we call it a "trouble spot" and wish we could get rid of it or shift it to areas where we need more padding. The "spot exercise" fallacy assumes, for example, that if you have fat deposits "pones" or "saddlebags" on the side of your hips, exercising the muscles underlying that fat will make it go away. Some not very scientific observations in the late 1800s are probably responsible for this misconception but more recent, careful investigations show that when we exercise, fuel comes from the bloodstream, and the body, acting as a composite unit, mobilizes fat from all over the body. The contracting muscle has no direct connection with the overlying adipose layer and does not get its energy from that particular piece of blubber.

General exercises are just as effective as "spot exercises" to remove fat. Any exercise burns calories (fat) and the fat comes from all over the body. One study showed that there is a tendency to lose more fat from the areas that are fattest. When someone says, "When I lose weight, I lose it in the wrong places; I always lose it from my face where I need it least," the truth of the matter is, they probably lose it from all over, but a fourth of an inch is more noticeable when lost from the face than it is when lost from the waist or hips. Local exercises are good to develop strength and endurance in specific muscle groups and do burn calories; *they do not selectively reduce fat deposits.*

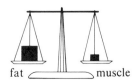

FIGURE 7.1 A pound of fat and a pound of lean

Fallacy 4: *Bumping fat body parts against the floor or wall will help reduce the fat.*

Bumping, thumping, massaging, rolling, vibrating, and shaking body parts are forms of passive exercise. To be useful for girth reduction, an exercise must make the muscle contract. When it does so, calories are burned and fat is mobilized. In addition, if an exercise is at the threshold of training, the muscle will get stronger and will experience hypertrophy (increase in size). Muscle tissue is more compact than fat. A pound of fat takes up more room than a pound of muscle, so that increasing lean body mass while decreasing fat means a loss in inches if weight remains constant (see Figure 7.1). Finally, strong, firm muscles can hold the body parts in positions of good posture, to give a slimmer appearance. Weak muscles in any area—hips, thighs, waist, arms—lead to a condition called flabbiness, and strengthening those specific muscles can change the body contour.

Fallacy 5: *Exercise can get rid of wrinkles and sagging skin.*

There is a phenomenon experienced with the aging process called "atrophy," in which body tissues begin to deterioriate. Proper exercise tends to delay the process in some tissues, but there is one physique problem that can not be altered by exercise. At about middle age, the subcutaneous tissues (those just under the skin) begin to atrophy noticeably and the skin loses its elasticity and seems to hang in flaps. It is what makes the jaw line sag, and jowls and wrinkles develop. Other common cosmetic problems are the flapping of the backs of the upper arms and the sagging of the seat. Face lifts and other plastic surgery procedures can remove these tell-tale marks of aging, but exercise is very limited in its effectiveness. It can **not** put elasticity back into the skin that has lost it nor build up atrophied subcutaneous tissues. It can **not** remove wrinkles nor get rid of stretch marks nor skin flaps. Exercise can firm up (strengthen) flabby muscles and add a little bulk to fill out sagging skin. And it can help improve fitness and health of the aging person so that they feel and act younger.

REFERENCES

1. Dietrich, J. and Waggoner, S., *The Complete Health Club Handbook,* New York, Simon and Schuster, 1983.
2. Lindsey, R., *A Survey and Critical Analysis of Practices Found in Selected Commercial Reducing Salons,* unpublished ms., Stillwater: Oklahoma State University Library, 1971.

Posture: Static and Dynamic

8

PRETEST

1. What are postural defects?
2. What constitutes proper body alignment when standing and when sitting?
3. What are the characteristics of a posture efficient chair?
4. What is an efficient walk?

The position in which you hold your body while lying, sitting, standing, or moving is called *posture*. Three things contribute to better posture and good health: a sufficient amount of sleep, proper exercise, and a balanced diet.

For the truth about your posture—ask your mirror; or better yet, have someone take a posture picture of you. On Chart XI in the Appendix, you will find places to attach your posture pictures. Underneath the pictures, your instructor can check your postural defects and give you an overall rating of them. Most of these defects are discussed in this unit.

Some of the factors conducive to poor posture are fatigue, obesity, self consciousness (e.g., disguising one's height by slumping), occupational conditions, (e.g., mail carrier with a heavy mail bag), and faulty habits. Bending over a low sink while washing dishes (working surfaces should be at elbow height), and watching TV or studying while sitting in a poor position are examples of faulty postural habits.

POSTURAL DEFECTS

Everyone has imperfections, but many of them are functional in nature and can be corrected or improved. Other conditions are structural and may require surgery to correct or improve.

1. **Round Shoulders**—Tips of the shoulders held forward. (This is usually accompanied by a forward head, sunken chest, and protruding scapulae.)
2. **Scoliosis**—Lateral curvature of the spine. This may be a very serious deformity and it requires referral to a physician. See figure 8.2.
3. **Lordosis**—Increased hyperextension in the lumbar region ("sway back"). See figure 8.1.

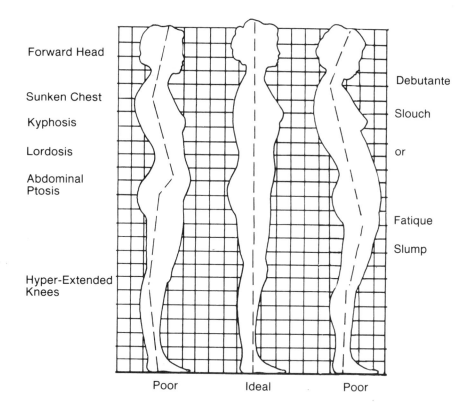

Forward Head

Sunken Chest

Kyphosis

Lordosis

Abdominal
Ptosis

Hyper-Extended
Knees

Debutante

Slouch

or

Fatique
Slump

Poor   Ideal   Poor

FIGURE 8.1 Good and bad posture: Side view

4. **Abdominal Ptosis**—Protruding abdomen (often accompanies lordosis). See figure 8.1.
5. **Kyphosis**—Round upper back ("hump back"). See figure 8.1.
6. **Flat Back**—Decreased spinal curvature or not enough curve, especially in the lower back.
7. **Hyperextended Knees**—Knees thrown back in a locked position. This habit often causes lordosis. See figure 8.1.
8. **Protruding Scapulae**—Protruding shoulder blades, or "wings."
9. **Body Lean**—A body shift from the ankles, either too far forward or backward.
10. **Forward Head**—Head thrust forward ("poke neck"). See figure 8.1.
11. **Sunken Chest**—Low or depressed chest. See figure 8.1.
12. **Fatigue Slump**—Hips thrust forward; trunk leaning backward; spinal flexion extends into lumbar region, with hyperextension at the sacroiliac joint. See figure 8.1.

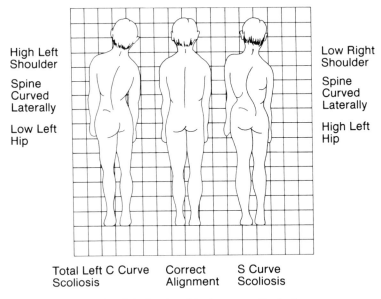

High Left
Shoulder

Spine
Curved
Laterally

Low Left
Hip

Low Right
Shoulder

Spine
Curved
Laterally

High Left
Hip

Total Left C Curve   Correct   S Curve
Scoliosis   Alignment   Scoliosis

FIGURE 8.2 Good and bad posture: Back view

WHY HAVE GOOD POSTURE

Perhaps the most obvious reason for obtaining good posture is that you will look better—and everyone wants to make a good *appearance.* Remember, the first impression you make upon a stranger is visual! A second reason is that *your clothes will probably fit better;* therefore, you will not have to wear loosely fitted clothes just to hide the "real you." A third reason for having good posture is that you will be more *efficient,* since joints, ligaments, and muscles will not be strained by poor posture and the range of movement will be greater. Finally, certain postural faults are linked to poor health. Lordosis probably makes one more susceptible to backache and dysmenorrhea; round shoulders and sunken chest may impair respiratory capacity; and head forward may lead to a variety of aches in the head, face, neck, and arms. Scoliosis will result in serious deformity and respiratory problems if not treated early, and a painful back will result.

PREREQUISITES FOR ACHIEVING GOOD POSTURE

1. You must have an *understanding* of what constitutes good posture.
2. You must have a *kinesthetic awareness* of where your body parts are in space.
3. You must have sufficient *muscle strength* for maintaining correct alignment.
4. You must have the *desire* to achieve good posture.
5. You must be *motivated* to practice good posture.

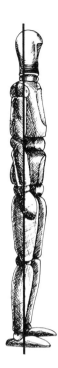

FIGURE 8.3 Good body alignment

CHARACTERISTICS OF PROPER BODY ALIGNMENT DURING STANDING

1. *The feet* should be parallel, slightly apart, with the weight balanced evenly on the heels, the outside borders, and the balls of the feet.
2. *The knees* should be straight and relaxed—neither bent nor hyperextended.
3. *The hips* should be tucked.
4. *The abdomen* should be flat.
5. *The chest* should be high but not exaggerated.
6. *The shoulders* should be neither forward, backward, nor elevated, but free and easy, with the shoulder blades flat.
7. *The head* should be centered over the trunk, with the *chin* level and the *ears* in line with the tips of the shoulders.
8. *The arms* should hang relaxed, with the palms of the hands facing the sides of the body.
9. *The back* should be neither too flat nor too curved.

If each body segment is balanced, a vertical line (gravity line) should extend from behind the ear, through the center of the shoulder and hip, behind the kneecap, and just in front of the ankle. Whenever one part moves out of line, the center of gravity shifts in the direction of movement of that segment, and another segment must adjust in the opposite direction to bring the center of gravity back over the base. A body is balanced when its center of gravity is over its supporting base. When wearing high heeled shoes or boots, the center of gravity should be adjusted at the ankles without disturbing the alignment of the various segments. If the backward adjustment is made at the waist, as is frequently the case, the entire alignment is affected and strain is felt in the lower back. The same principle is true in counterbalancing the added weight in pregnancy or when carrying an object.

Muscles work in pairs, and both must be exercised in order not to have postural faults. For example, strengthening the chest muscles could cause round shoulders and sunken chest unless the upper back muscles are also strengthened. If your body segments are not in alignment, you may need to strengthen weak muscle groups and stretch tight or short muscle groups by the use of special exercise. The maintenance of proper posture depends upon sufficient muscular endurance. Muscular endurance is the ability of a muscle to perform work for a sustained period. Muscles which fatigue easily will be unable to maintain correct body alignment.

Most of us need reminders to aid us in achieving good posture. These key words might be helpful.

1. *Stand tall.*
2. *Sit tall.*
3. *Walk tall.*
4. *Think tall.*

SITTING AND RISING

Much of your day is spent sitting. You sit to eat, study, work, and socialize. You sit in class, in a theater, in church, and at an athletic event. Not only should your sitting posture be good, but the act of getting into and out of the seated position should be performed gracefully and efficiently.

Sitting In and Rising from a Chair

As you enter a room, choose the chair best suited to you. Ideally, a chair should have arms, be low enough to allow you to place your feet on the floor while keeping your knees above hip level, and be shallow enough for your back to be placed against the chair back. Seat backs are best if hard or firmly padded, not soft. They should contact the back four to six inches above the seat.

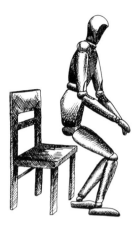

FIGURE 8.4 Proper mechanics of sitting and rising

Approach the chair at a slight angle from the right or left, and touch the center front of the chair with the calf of your leg as you turn your back to it. The foot nearest the chair should be well under it, with your weight on both feet. Keep your neck and head in line with your trunk and your trunk erect, with the hips tucked under as you bend at the hips and knees and incline your body slightly forward. Shift your body weight to your rear foot, as your body is lowered into the chair, by using the leg muscles. Keep your pelvis under your trunk, your feet under your pelvis, and transfer the body weight gradually and smoothly.

Certain types of chairs present problems. More muscular effort is needed if the seat is low. If the seat is deep, the hands may be placed on the chair arms to help retain balance, but try to avoid using the arms to lower your body.

Sit on the whole chair—if a "scoot" is necessary, try to move back in one attempt. Sit on the two knob-like pelvic bones (tuberosities of the ischia); hold the head and chest erect, with the abdomen in; lean against the back rest; and relax your shoulders. Women, should cross their legs above the knee or at the ankle. Some women prefer to place the heel of one foot against the instep of the other foot, keeping the knees together.

To rise, simply reverse the sitting procedure. If it is necessary to "scoot" forward, try to do it in one attempt. Place one foot as far back under the chair as possible. Lean slightly forward from the hips, keeping your hips tucked under and your chest and head erect. Push up by extending the knee of the rear foot as you shift your weight from the rear foot to the front foot. Use your thigh muscles to "press into the floor" by pushing on your heels. Your hands may be placed on the arms of the chair to help you retain your balance, but do not push up with them.

When driving on long trips, move the seat forward so that your knees are above the level of your hips. If the seat does not support the lower back, slip a pillow behind it. During long sitting periods, bulging wallets in the back pocket can press on the sciatic nerve sending shooting pains down the leg.

WALKING

You should walk the way you stand—with a well-balanced, relaxed, and poised body alignment. The purpose in walking is to move forward; therefore, there should be no wasted motion in the lateral plane. Limit the motion to arms and legs with a minimum of trunk movement.

Stand in your best posture. Swing your leg straight ahead, keeping your knee flexed, with the major movement flowing from the hip. Point your toes straight ahead. Place the heel of your foot very lightly on the floor; transfer your weight to the outer border and then the ball of the foot, "feel" the floor with your toes; and then push off with the big toe. Move the feet on parallel tracks, about two inches apart. Stride length will vary with the type of dress, leg length, and speed of your gait; but in general, it will be approximately the length of your foot. Let your arms swing freely and easily from the shoulder joint in opposition to your leg movements. The length of the swing depends on the length of the stride—just enough to keep your chest facing forward. The palm of your hand should face your leg, with finger tips just brushing lightly in passing.

Since there is no one best standing posture, there is no one best walking gait. Body structures and personalities vary and are expressed in an individual's walk. However, wide variation may need to be modified.

STAIR CLIMBING

Good body mechanics in ascending and descending stairs should be considered from the standpoints of safety, efficiency, and appearance. Several factors are important in regard to safety. Place your entire foot on the step to prevent arch strain and to help retain balance. Many steps are narrow, so it may be necessary to turn the body slightly sideways in order to place the entire foot on the tread. Glance occasionally at several steps ahead of you; however, do not look at your feet. You should use the handrail to help retain balance by sliding the hand lightly along the rail.

When ascending stairs, the body should be lifted forward and upward with the leg of your *forward* foot. The knee is bent as your foot is placed on the step, and is extended with the strong thigh (quadriceps) muscles as the weight is transferred to the lead foot. When descending, the knee is bent, and the body weight is supported by the strong thigh muscles (again using the quadriceps) of the *rear* leg as the weight is transferred to the lead foot.

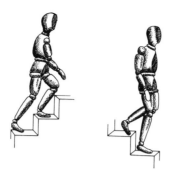

FIGURE 8.5 Proper mechanics when ascending and descending stairs

Your posture should be erect. Carry your head and chest high, and avoid pushing the hips backward when taking each step. Watch where you are going by occasionally focusing your eyes on the steps ahead without jutting your head forward. Move your body smoothly and steadily in a gliding manner. A jerky bounce can be avoided by using the knees as "shock absorbers," keeping them slightly bent and not straightening them on every step.

SELECTED EXERCISES FOR POSTURAL FAULTS

Abdominal Ptosis

(These exercises are also good for lordosis.)

Cat-Backs (strengthens abdominals). On hands and knees permit the abdominals "to droop" and the back to sway. Then flatten the abdomen by "pulling it in," and "hump" the back, holding for a count of five. Relax for five counts and repeat five times.

Pelvic Tilt (strengthens abdominals). An isometric exercise done in a supine position, with the knees bent and slightly apart. Press the spine down on the floor and hold it while contracting the abdominals and gluteals. Hold for ten counts, and relax. Repeat five times.

Crunches (*Partial Sit-ups*) (strengthens abdominals). Refer to chapter 1 "Tests for Physical Fitness." When performed for the purpose of abdominal strengthening, it is best to leave the feet free and unsupported. This helps to ensure that the proper muscles are performing the work and avoids strain on the back.

Lordosis

Wall Exercise (strengthens abdominals and stretches the lower back). Stand with your back to the wall and the heels an inch from the wall. Flatten the lower back against the wall and walk away maintaining the flattened back. Return to the wall and check to see if you have kept that position.

Knee Raise (stretches lower back). Lie in supine position. Bend one knee and bring it to the chest, grasp behind the knee and pull it to the chest, then hold for a count of ten. Alternate right and left legs. Repeat four times with each leg.

Round Shoulders, Sunken Chest, Kyphosis, and Protruding Scapulae

Corner Exercise (stretches pectorals). Stand in a corner, with the arms bent at the elbows (shoulder level) and parallel with the floor. With the hands against opposite walls, lean into the corner. Repeat five times.

Arm Circles (increases strength or endurance of muscles in upper back and shoulders and stretches pectorals; also for forward head). Arms raised sideward to shoulder level, with *palms up* circle backward four times; then bend the arms at the elbows and push backward, bringing the shoulder blades together. Keep the chin tucked and the neck extended; do not allow the head to thrust forward. Repeat eight to twenty-five times.

Prone Arm Raise (increases strength or endurance of muscles in upper back and shoulders). Lie in a prone position, with the arms extended forward. Raise arms straight toward the ceiling—first left, then right, then both. Keep your forehead in contact with the floor. Repeat the three movements five to twenty-five times.

Back Stroke (increases strength or endurance of muscles in upper back and shoulders). Sit or stand. Place the back of the right hand on the right side of the face; press the elbow straight back. Keeping the elbow back, reach backwards with the right hand. Alternate left and right five to twenty-five times on each side, as in swimming the back crawl.

Forward Head

Wall Press (strengthens neck muscles). Stand with your back to the wall with the heels two or three inches from the wall. Press the back of your head against the wall, keep the chin down, and do not increase the lumbar curve. Hold for a count of four, relax for five counts, and repeat three or four times.

Finger Press (strengthens neck muscles). Sit. Interlace the fingers behind the head. Pull forward with the arms as you push back with the head. Hold for a count of five, relax for five counts, and repeat three or four times.

Head Lift (strengthens neck muscles). Lie in a prone position, with hands clasped behind the head. Apply slight resistance with hands while raising head from the floor. Hold for a count of five, then relax. Repeat five times.

Scoliosis*

(S curve with left dorsal and right lumbar curves. If curves are opposite, reverse the exercise position.)

Bar Hang (stretching). Hang from rings or a bar by the hands with the arms fully extended.

Prone Stretch. Lie prone. Stretch the right arm over head and at the same time stretch the left arm downward and across the back. Hold this position for 30 seconds.

Supine Stretch. Lie supine. Draw both knees to the chest and clasp the hands around the thighs. Hold this position for 30 seconds.

Scoliosis*

(C curve to the left. If the curve is to the right, reverse the exercises.)

Bar Hang. (see Scoliosis, S curve.)

Stretch Down. Stand with the hands on the hips. Stretch the left arm down at the side and push down firmly. Do not bend the body toward the left side. Repeat five or six times.

Overhead Stretch. Stand with the hands on the hips. Stretch the right arm up overhead; press the left hand against the rib cage at a point which forces the spine into a straighter position. Repeat five or six times.

Flat Back

Shoulder Lift (strengthens muscles in lower back). Lie prone. Place the hands behind the neck, raise the shoulders off the floor, arch the back, keep the hips in contact with the floor. Repeat five or six times.

Lumbar Arch (strengthens muscles in lower back). Stand. Interlock the fingers behind the back in the lumbar area. Press the elbows down and back; try to bring the elbows together. Arch the back in the lumbar area.

*If you have scoliosis see your physician and perform these exercises only with physician approval.

Care of the Back and Body Mechanics in Daily Living

9

PRETEST

1. What is lordosis?
2. How do you prevent back problems?
3. What are selected exercises that may be done to alleviate back pain?
4. What is the correct way to lift and carry?

The spine must support much of the body weight as well as absorb shock and provide for a wide range of trunk movements. These functions are made possible by a flexible backbone composed of 24 separate vertebrae plus the sacrum and coccyx, with discs of cartilage between them to absorb shock and prevent friction. While such an arrangement does allow for weight bearing and movement, this same architecture makes the back susceptible to strain and injury. "Oh, my aching back!" is a common complaint that afflicts an estimated 8 million Americans sometime during their lives! It is one of the nation's most expensive health problems and next to headaches, is probably the most common painful affliction.

According to many authorities, at the rate back pain is increasing, more people will suffer from chronic and recurrent back problems than from any other single medical ailment. Ninety-five percent of all backaches occur in the lower spine. This area sustains the greatest stress from bending and improper posture during sitting and standing.

CAUSES OF BACKACHES

There are many causes of backaches. Some are actually unrelated to the back, such as kidney disease, peptic ulcer, tipped uterus, infection of the ovaries, or gallbladder. Some problems may be caused by hereditary structures. Backaches are sometimes psychosomatic—for example, backaches can be a reaction to stress. Stressful situations may stimulate the adrenal glands, creating a change in the body chemistry causing muscle spasms.

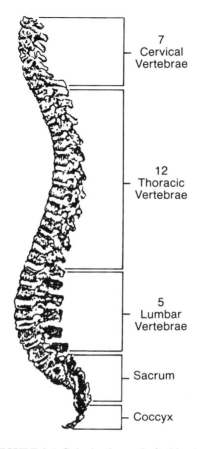

7
Cervical
Vertebrae

12
Thoracic
Vertebrae

5
Lumbar
Vertebrae

Sacrum

Coccyx

FIGURE 9.1 Spinal column: Left side view

Other causes include arthritis, fatigue produced by malnutrition, muscular weakness resulting from inactivity, muscle strain from sudden or forceful bending or twisting, unequal leg lengths, and osteoporosis. Osteoporosis is a condition in which the spine becomes porous and brittle due to the loss of calcium. This occurs mainly in women during the postmenopausal period because of a hormone imbalance, but it may also occur in men. It is not unusual to see disc problems in the early teens, because rapid growth in childhood may cause the spine to outgrow its muscular support.

Low Back Pain

The most frequent causes of lower backaches are fatigue and strain due to improper use of the back in daily activities, such as lifting too heavy an object or incorrect lifting. Poor posture often is a contributing factor—especially swayback. A swayed back (lordosis) is particularly vulnerable to strain and subject to herniated disc due to the excessive curvature of the lumbar portion of the spine.

As Americans become more sedentary in an increasingly automated society, their backs become more vulnerable to injury. The risks are greater for sedentary persons than for the active laborers; for example, the woman who stops exercising when she becomes pregnant will be more prone to backache because her abdominal muscles will become weak.

The head-forward position places strain on the posterior neck muscles and can lead to such symptoms as headaches, cricks, dizziness, and pain reflected in the face, scalp, arms, and chest. Neck strain can contribute to pain in the thoracic and lumbar spine.

Upper Back and Neck Pain

Many people have hypersensitive spots in their upper back and shoulder muscles which can become very painful and may cause pain to be referred to other areas of the body. Tension headache may result from this referred pain. The hypersensitive spots are called *trigger points*. Tense persons and those who assume static postures for long periods of time (such as typists or students) are very prone to these. Some stretching exercises are included in this chapter to help prevent or relieve these "knots" in your muscles.

PREVENTION AND TREATMENT

To prevent back and neck problems, avoid strain from poor posture and improper use of the back, and on the positive side, perform strengthening and stretching exercises such as those described in this chapter. The chief support for the lower back is the *abdominal muscles*. These must be strengthened along with all other muscles which aid in good posture; these include the *gluteals*—the buttock muscles. The abdominals pull the pelvis up in front and the gluteals pull the pelvis down in back, reducing pelvic tilt. The *back extensor muscles* provide posterior support, while the *lateral trunk muscles* provide lateral support and motion.

It is important that you understand that these four muscle groups work together and are essential to the proper function of the back. Your preventive exercises should be designed to strengthen these muscles and should be done regularly to maintain them. (See chapter 4 for additional abdominal and gluteal exercises.)

Those who have lordosis should stretch the muscles in the lumbar region and stretch the hip flexors. For those with low back problems, toe touches should be done in a sitting rather than a standing position, so as to reduce the momentum of the upper body.

Those who have lumbar kyphosis (flat back) and a backward tilted pelvis, may need to strengthen the lower back muscles and stretch the hamstrings and gluteals to restore the normal curvature.

When the problem appears to be moderate muscle strain of the lower back, rest, heat, and aspirin usually bring relief. If the pain has not subsided in two or three days, seek the advice of a physician, preferably an orthopedic specialist. The only cure for a "conventional" bad back, once the original cause is diagnosed and corrected, is physical reconditioning. Exercise can be the tool for rebuilding the back structure. This will mean daily exercise; 15 minutes twice daily is preferred. Start slowly and avoid overdoing at the beginning.

Muscle relaxants can be prescribed for temporary relief, but they do not remove the cause. Lying on a hard floor sometimes helps to relieve the pain. There are also times when complete bed rest is necessary. Exercise or activities may be prescribed by physicians. Swimming may be a good exercise, since the buoyancy of the body in the water removes stress on the back. The crawl and the side strokes are the best; avoid the butterfly because of the jerking motion of the spine.

Guidelines for the Prevention of Back Problems

The following suggestions are guidelines to help you prevent back and neck strain.

1. Avoid the swayback position at all times by taking such precautions as the following:
   a. During prolonged standing, prop one foot on a stool, bar, or rail, and alternate the foot which takes the major load. Circulate; do not stand in one place for extended periods of time.
   b. When sitting, keep one or both knees higher than the hips by crossing the legs (above the knees) or using a foot rest, keeping the knees bent.
   c. When lying, keep the knees and hips bent; avoid lying on the abdomen; and when lying on the back, place a pillow or lift under the knees.

   d. When lifting and carrying objects, attempting to move a load which is too heavy, or lifting with a jerk, could cause a hernia (rupture).

   e. When driving a car, a lumbar pad is recommended to maintain the normal curve. Keeping the knees at or above the hip level will prevent lordosis and relieve stress on the back. Get out of the car every hour or two and walk around for a few minutes. If the tilt of the seat can be altered, change the angle periodically.

2. Prevent neck strain by avoiding the head-forward position. The forward thrust is apt to occur in such activities as card playing, sewing, and studying. Sleeping on a high pillow or reclining while watching TV will also result in neck strain.

3. Try to resist wearing high-heeled shoes or boots. They tend to tilt the pelvis, throwing the spine out of line. If you must wear them, do so for only short periods of time.

4. Be aware of how you carry your wallet or purse. Sitting on a thick wallet in the hip pocket can press on the sciatic nerve. Carrying a heavy purse habitually on the same side of the body can result in neck, shoulder, and back pain.

5. Do general exercises involving the entire body to avoid having weak muscles.

6. Get adequate rest, and avoid pushing yourself mentally or physically to the point of overfatigue.

7. When doing activities that may aggravate your back (such as painting overhead or cleaning high shelves) rotate among the tasks to avoid prolonged strain on one particular area.

In addition to the above suggestions, you can help avoid backache by such common-sense practices as "warming up" before engaging in strenuous activity, sleeping on a firm mattress, stretching occasionally to relieve tension while studying at a desk, and avoid sudden, jerky movements of the back. It will also help if you keep your weight down to normal, and observe the rules for good body mechanics described throughout this book.

BODY MECHANICS IN DAILY LIVING

Lifting, carrying, pushing, and pulling are normal, everyday activities. It is important to perform them in a correct manner in order to be more efficient, while protecting joints and muscles from undue strain. The avoidance of strain, especially of the back, is the prime consideration in these activities. Some suggestions are given below to aid you in attaining this objective.

Lifting and Carrying

Improper methods of lifting and carrying may cause strain, especially to the lower back. The best method of lifting and carrying a given object will depend upon its weight, mass, and shape. However, the following principles for *lifting* are applicable at all times:

1. Stand close to the object, either in a forward-stride position, with the object at the side, or a side-stride position, with the object between the knees. In the side-stride position, the object is closer to the center of gravity and the lift is straight upward. (See figures 9.2 and 9.3.)
2. Keep your back erect, and bend at the hips and knees.
3. Lower your body only as far as necessary, directly downward.
4. Grasp the object and lift with your leg muscles by extending the legs, keeping the object close to your body. Do not lift with a "jerk."
5. Reverse the procedure when lowering the object. Do not twist as you extend the spine.

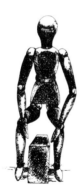

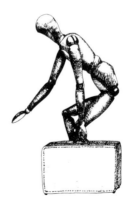

FIGURE 9.2 Lifting object in front of body

FIGURE 9.3 Lifting object at side of body

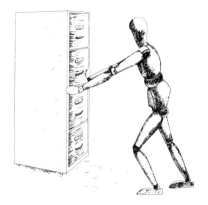

FIGURE 9.4 Pushing a large, heavy object

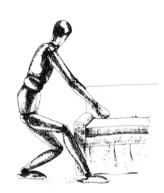

FIGURE 9.5 Pulling a large, heavy object

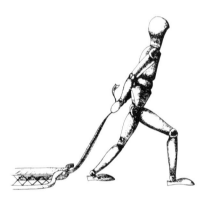

FIGURE 9.6 Pulling a low object by adding a longer handle

6. Push or pull heavy objects, if this can be done efficiently, rather than lifting them. A good guideline for women is to lift no more than one-third of their body weight. Men should generally lift no more than one-half their body weight. (See figures 9.4, 9.5, 9.6.)

Some suggestions for *carrying* objects are:

1. Keep the object close to the body's center of gravity.
2. Divide the load, if possible, carrying half in each arm.
3. If the load cannot be divided, occasionally alternate the load from one side of the body to the other.

4. Extend the opposite arm for balance, or lean away from the load.
5. When carrying books—a common activity for students—some faults to be *avoided* are:
   a. Always carrying books on the same side. This tends to cause the shoulder to be higher than the other and may lead to scoliosis.
   b. Carrying the books in front of the chest. You may have a tendency to lean back to compensate for the additional weight or to hunch forward as you wrap your arms around the books. These actions make the posture unattractive and place a strain on the back.

      Preferably, books should be carried in a brief case or back pack and should be divided equally between both arms. The principles for carrying books also apply when carrying the baby, laundry, grocery sacks, and other loads.
6. Some cautions for *lifting* and *carrying* are:
   a. Do not try to lift or carry loads too heavy for you.
   b. To minimize lower back strain, do not lift or carry heavy objects higher than waist level, except when carrying on the shoulder or head.

Pulling and Pushing (See figures 9.4, 9.5, 9.6)

The best method for *pushing* or *pulling* a given object will depend upon its weight, mass, resistance, and shape, but some general tips are:

1. Keep the back as straight as possible.
2. Use a wide base for balance (stride position).
3. Grasp the object firmly, with the arms fully extended.
4. Bend at the hips and knees, letting the leg muscles do the work.
5. Alternate muscles used by changing the direction you face, such as backward, forward, or sideward.
6. Lean forward from the ankles so that the center of gravity is ahead of the pushing foot.
7. Put glass or metal coasters under heavy furniture to ease the task where friction is great.
8. "Walk" objects too heavy to be moved, such as a refrigerator or couch, by applying force alternately, at one end then the other, in a rotating ("walking") motion.
9. Pull a low object with a long handle or rope to make the task easier (see figure 9.6).

Practicing proper body mechanics in the daily tasks mentioned in the preceding paragraphs will not only help you to avoid strain but will help you to conserve energy for other activities.

SELECTED BACK EXERCISES

Also see abdominal exercises, chapter 4 and relaxation exercises, chapter 11. These exercises are more effective after a period of relaxation.

To Strengthen Upper Back

Also see exercises for the back on pages 62 and 63.

Prone Back Lift—Lie prone (face down), with hands clasped behind your neck. Pull your shoulder blades together, raising the elbows off the floor. Slowly raise your head and chest off the floor by arching the upper back. Hold this position for three seconds, then slowly return to the starting position. Repeat 10 times. Caution: *do not* arch the lower back; lift only until the sternum (breastbone) clears the floor.

Isometric Push Back—Tailor sit or stand, with the head up, chin in, elbows raised to shoulder level, fingertips placed on the back of the neck. Push the head and neck backward; and push the fingertips forward, as the elbows are forced backward to flatten the upper back. Hold for five or six seconds, and then relax. Repeat two or three times per day.

To Strengthen Lower Back

Not desirable for those with lordosis.

Kneeling Leg Lift—Kneeling with head resting on hands, raise one leg until it is in line with the body. Do not allow the back to arch. **Note:** As a general rule, it is best to avoid arching (hyperextending) the lower back during exercises, especially for those with lordosis. Repeat 10 to 20 times alternating legs.

Limb Lift—Lie in a prone position, with the arms extended overhead and with the legs straight. Slowly lift an arm and leg on the same side of the body. *Do not* arch the back. Hold for three or four seconds, and lower slowly to the starting position. Do not roll the body away from the side that is lifted. Alternating sides, repeat eight times.

To Stretch Lower Back and Alleviate Low Back Pain

Also see exercises for lordosis, page 122.

Lumbar Stretch—Lie supine (on the back), with knees bent and the feet flat on the floor near your buttocks. Contract your abdominal muscles, flattening the lower back against the floor. Draw one knee up, grasp the thigh and pull it down tightly against your chest with your arms. Return to the starting position, then repeat with the other leg. Repeat with each leg 10 to 20 times. When this exercise becomes easy, progress to raising both knees at the same time. For an even greater stretch, try to pull the knees to the axillae (armpits). Combine lumbar stretching with abdominal-strengthening exercises to alleviate low back pain and lordosis.

Rock-A-Bye—Lie supine, draw both knees to the chest, and wrap your arms around the thighs to bring them close to the trunk. Rock forward and backward as though you were trying to come to a sitting position. Rock four or five times, relax, and repeat three times.

Sit and Reach—Sit with the knees extended and the feet together. Reach forward and grasp your ankles, pulling the trunk forward; hold five seconds. Relax, and repeat three times. Do **not** "lock" your knees.

Sit and Curl—Sit in chair and bend forward and hug knees.

To Stretch Trigger Points in Upper Back and Neck

Neck Rotation—Point left fingers toward the rear, toward left ear and place palm of hand against jaw; push head toward right while resisting by trying to rotate head to left; hold isometrically for four seconds, then turn head right as far as possible and hold for four seconds. Perform exercise four times then repeat in other direction four times. Do this exercise four times daily.

Arm Stretch—Face wall and extend both arms forward to shoulder level, with fingers six to eight inches from wall. Swing the right arm down and around in a big circle, then reach as far forward as possible, trying to touch the wall with the right fingers, without turning your trunk. Hold four seconds. Repeat four times on each side, four times daily.

Rib Separator—Stand with weight on left foot and drop right hip; grasp hands above and behind the head. Bend upper trunk to left and use left arm to pull right arm to left as far as possible. Hold for four seconds. Repeat four times on each side, four times daily. You should feel a stretch under your arm and down the side of your ribs.

Care of the Feet

10

PRETEST

1. What factors should be considered in selecting a jogging shoe?
2. What are some common foot problems?
3. What causes foot problems?
4. How may most foot problems be prevented?
5. How can shin splints be prevented?

Do your feet hurt? If not, you probably have given very little thought to this part of your anatomy that you pick up and put down thousands of times each day, moves you a thousand or so miles each year, and serves as your base of support for about six hours each day. Approximately 80 percent of the adult population complain of foot problems. This is a startling figure since almost 99 percent of all feet are perfect at birth. Most of the problems can be prevented or cured by following some basic rules of health.

The foot is a complicated structure. Each foot contains 26 bones, 197 ligaments, 19 muscles (18 in the sole alone), and 33 joints. The 14 toe bones are called phalanges; the five bones that make up the midfoot are called metatarsals, and the seven irregular bones in the back of the foot are called tarsals. The main purposes of the feet are weight bearing and locomotion. The number of arches in the foot has been debated by different authorities as some say there are three, some four, while others contend only two. The most familiar is the longitudinal arch, which runs from the base of the first phalanx to the heel. (See Figures 10.1 and 10.2).

It functions as a weight carrier and a shock absorber. Many consider this arch as two separate arches—the inner and outer longitudinals. The metatarsal arch runs laterally across the ball of the foot and helps to give balance and absorb shock.

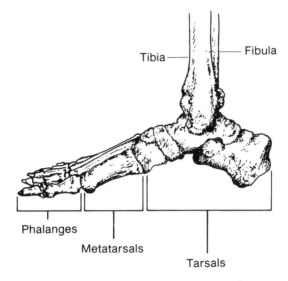

FIGURE 10.1 The foot: Side view

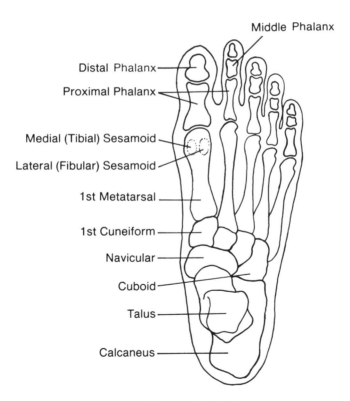

FIGURE 10.2 Bones of the foot

SELECTION OF FOOTWEAR

The majority of foot problems are caused by wearing improperly fitted shoes, shoes of the wrong type, or by not using the foot correctly. If the cause is improperly fitting shoes, the first step in combating the problem is to discard the shoes.

Shoes should never be handed down from person to person if a correct fit is desired. The two most common mistakes made in buying shoes are getting them too narrow or too short. Shoes should be at least a half-inch longer (thumb width) than the longest toe when standing and there should be room for the toes to spread out. The ball of the foot should be at the widest part of the shoe; the heel should be snug enough to not slip up and down. Try to buy shoes in the late afternoon, when the foot may be as much as a full size larger than it was early in the day. New shoes should be "broken-in" by wearing them for short periods before extended wear such as all day shopping trips. High heels change the center of gravity which puts strain on the metatarsal arch and tends to shorten the calf muscles. Leather shoes which lace are almost unbeatable for support. They hug the foot, give with the foot, absorb shock, and allow the foot to breathe.

Shoes are for protection, support, traction, cushioning from the ground, balance of foot deformities, and the accommodation of foot injuries. People with normal feet and no injuries are able to wear almost any type of shoes with no pain or disability; but if a person has recurrent problems, then certain types of shoes may help and other types of shoes may aggravate them. For instance, a runner who is susceptible to Achilles tendonitis requires a flexible shoe with cushioning of the bottom of the heel and good elevation. A person with weak ankles and instability needs a shoe that will provide support and balance at heel contact. Calluses on the bottom of the foot require good cushioning. Corns on the top of the foot require a deep toe box and proper fit.

ATHLETIC SHOES

Shoes are designed for a specific purpose; each kind of athletic shoe is designed for a particular activity to provide the correct support and stability. A jogging shoe should *not* be used for other sports activities because the elevated heel makes the foot slide forward in the shoe when doing quick stops (such as used in basketball and tennis). Also, rippled soles are better for jogging and running while the nubbed, plain, and herringbone soles are better suited for other activities.

Shoe Parts

The *outersole* (bottom) of the shoe provides the striking surface of the shoe. The *midsole* (second layer) provides shock dispersion and helps prevent shock-related injuries such as shin splints, stress fractures, and tendonitis. The *insole* is that part on which the foot directly rests. At the back of the shoe is the *heel*

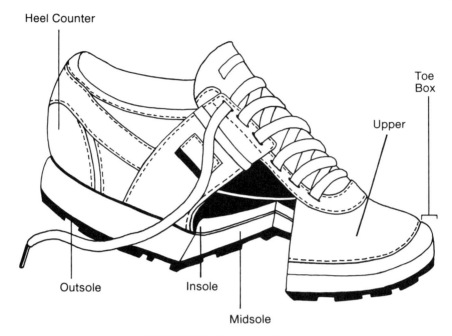

FIGURE 10.3 Key parts of a shoe

counter, a firm cup that holds your heel. It can be extended on the lateral or medial side of the shoe to give added support. At the front of the shoe is the *toe box* which should be wide and deep to provide for comfort.

Jogging Shoes

Shoes are the only major equipment investment essential for the jogger. They have a more direct effect on the pleasure, performance, and health of the runner than any other factor, including training, since a runner cannot train freely on painful feet. You need to know the difference between good shoes and merely pretty ones.

Runner's World issues a shoe edition each October where different shoes are evaluated. They emphasize four basics: stability, cushioning, outsole durability and good fit. They suggest that you consider the following features when buying running shoes![1,2]

1. *Shape*—The three different shapes are straight, semicurved, and curved. The straighter the shoe, the more support it will give.

2. *Construction*—The options are board-lasted, slip-lasted and combination-lasted. In general, board-lasted shoes are the most stable and are intended for overpronators while slip-lasted are the most flexible. Combination-lasted attempts to provide both stability and comfort.

3. *Midsole*—It is the most important component in a running shoe. All midsole designs strive for cushioning, stability, and durability.

4. *Outsole*—The harder the outsole, the longer it will wear and the heavier it will be.

5. *Insole*—This part of the shoe is made of a cushiony material (the high tech favorite of the late 1980s is polyurethane) and is often contoured to support the shape of the foot, particularly at the arch. Some are lined with terry cloth to absorb perspiration and to reduce slippage.

6. *Heel Counter*—The cup in the back of the shoe upper helps to control excessive foot motion.

7. *Fit*—The shoe must fit your foot, biomechanically as well as in terms of comfort. If you have flat feet, you will do best with a straight shoe which will provide medial support. Runners with high arches usually find the curved design most appropriate, because of the lateral support. Most companies have changed their lacing system to provide a better fit, but in 1987 only one company manufactured different widths.

Aerobic Shoes

An aerobic shoe can be too flexible or too stiff. The shoe must flex in the forefoot region while giving lateral and medial support for good motion control. A good aerobic shoe has a soft resilient midsole to aid in shock dispersion. It should have a sturdy heel counter to hold the foot in place. If you have a high arch and do high intensity aerobics, shock absorption should be at the top of your list. If you have flat feet and overpronate, look for stability. Test your shoes before buying by jumping and doing a few steps and turns. Roll up on the balls of your feet to see if your heel slips out of the shoe. If this occurs, the shoe is probably too stiff. Do not rely on standard sizing but allow about a half-inch space between the longest toe and the end of the shoe.

Court Shoes

In sports such as basketball, volleyball, racquetball, and tennis, the shoe's sole is the most important element. The tread design should offer forward and lateral stopping, balance, stability, and traction. Tennis needs a durable sole because of court surfaces and grooved tread should be selected for traction. Court activities need a shoe that has the ability to disperse shock and have motion control to prevent ankle turns. Leather uppers are good for court games because of their breathability and support. When purchasing leather uppers, the fit should be slightly snug as leather will stretch.

Walking Shoes

There are two basic types—power-walking and fitness-walking. The features to look for are about the same except, generally, the fitness-walking shoe is more lightweight than the power-walking one and will not hold up as well under fast-paced, heavy mileage. When buying either, look for those that feel good on your feet, have a flexible forefoot, and allow your foot to spread when it bears your body weight. Too, the shoe must offer stability, have a well-cushioned heel, and have a durable outsole that provides necessary traction. For trail walking, ankle-high boots are good.

COMMON FOOT PROBLEMS

You can prevent or minimize most foot problems by wearing the correct style of shoe, ones that fit properly, and by following some simple rules.

1. Walk properly. One should contact the ground first with the heel, then the outer border of the foot, then the ball of the foot, and finally push off with the toes. Toes should point straight ahead. Toeing out (slue foot) may lead to pronation.
2. Wear well-fitting socks and hosiery to prevent friction, to absorb shock, and to absorb perspiration avoid stretch socks. Make sure that they give your toes room to wiggle but not fit so loosely that they wrinkle. Change them at least once a day.
3. Keep your feet clean and dry.
4. Lubricate your skin, except between the toes, with lotion or cream. If your feet perspire alot, dust them with foot powder or cornstarch.
5. Inspect your feet regularly for small injuries, red spots, fungus infections, blisters and plantar warts.
6. Change shoes frequently; do not wear the same pair every day. If the shoes are not comfortable, do not wear them.
7. Keep your shoes in good shape. Replace worn heels and do not let the soles become too thin. If the lining becomes worn, it is time to discard the shoes.

In addition to proper footwear, proper use of the feet, and foot exercises, it may be necessary for some people to have corrective devices (orthotics) prescribed by the physician or podiatrist to alleviate certain foot problems.

Some common foot problems are:

Hard and Soft Corns. Corns, small areas of thickened dead skin, are caused by improperly fitting shoes and hose. They can often be relieved by corn pads, or in the case of a soft corn, the use of lamb's wool between the toes. If the corns persist, see your physician or podiatrist (a person who specializes in treating diseases, injuries, and defects of the feet). Do not be a bathroom surgeon; never use corn salves or drops because the caustic acid may injure the surrounding skin.

Calluses. Calluses, like corns, are accumulations of thickened dead skin that protect against friction and pressure but form as thick flat pads on weight bearing areas of the heel and sole. They are caused by friction due to improperly fitting shoes. We sometimes find "loafer's knots" on the heel resulting from loosely fitting shoes rubbing the area. To prevent, wear properly fitting shoes, use cushioned inner soles, and lubricate your feet with cream or lotion. If the callus is uncomfortable, seek medical advice.

Bunions. A chronic inflammation of the bursa sac, bunions are usually found on the joint of the first phalanx. This is caused by pressure and rubbing of the shoe and is aggravated by short, pointed shoes, short or stretch hose, and high heels. Bunions can be relieved by wearing wider shoes, preferably of soft leather. Surgical correction is sometimes necessary because the toe becomes partially dislocated (Hallux Valgus).

Ingrown Toenails. Ingrown toenails are the result of cutting the toenails curved instead of straight across, and of improperly fitting shoes and hose. The nail cuts into the skin causing pain and the possibility of infection. This condition usually requires professional care.

Athlete's Foot. Athlete's foot is a fungus infection which usually appears between the toes. It thrives under warm, moist conditions, so the best prevention is to keep the feet clean, dry, and powdered. Wash your feet twice a day, change your shoes and hose/socks at least once a day, and wear open shoes when possible. Rubber thongs can help to protect your feet in public bathing or swimming areas. Medication for treatment is available in powder, ointment, or spray.

Blisters. Blisters are fluid-filled cushions that form when the outer skin layer (epidermis) is damaged by friction from shoes or socks. To prevent them, wear well-fitting shoes and socks, keep your feet dry, and eliminate the cause of the friction. If a shoe rubs your foot, rub a lubricant on the spot and cover it with a bandage. Let small blisters break on their own. If they break, cleanse with soap and water. See a doctor if the blister does not heal.

Crooked or Overlapping Toes. Deformed toes may result from wearing shoes that are too short or narrow and hose that are too short or of the stretch type. Sometimes, toe deformities are congenital in origin.

Bromidrosis. Bromidrosis is excessive perspiration and odor. Use the same prevention as for athlete's foot. Avoid prolonged wearing of canvas shoes. Antiperspirant deodorant sprays or powder may be helpful.

Plantar Warts. These painful growths that appear on the soles of the feet are caused by a virus and may be transmitted from place to place and person to person. They should be treated by a physician or podiatrist.

Poor Circulation and Fatigue. Poor circulation and fatigue result from long standing and strenuous use. Some relief may be obtained by elevating the feet, massaging the feet and using contrast baths.

Shortened Achilles Tendon. A shortened Achilles tendon ("heel cord") is caused by constant wearing of high heels, which makes it uncomfortable to wear "flats." The means of correction is to stretch the tendon through exercise (see exercises on pages 142–143).

Heel Pain (Plantar fasciitis). Most physicians believe the pain comes from inflammation or a tear in the plantar fascia on the bottom of the foot at the point where it attaches to the heel. This is caused by constant impact and overuse. The best treatment is rest but using shock absorbent heel pads and a firm heel cup may help.

WEAK FOOT CONDITION

Some symptoms of weak feet are pain in the arch, calf, and lower back; pronation; and general fatigue. Pronation occurs when the weight is borne on the inner border of the foot. The longitudinal arch is lowered, the inner ankle bone protrudes, and the Achilles tendon fails to retain the normal vertical line.

Slight pronation is a natural part of foot movement as this movement helps absorb some of the force of impact. However, excessive pronation is a serious problem. The primary cause of running injuries is excessive pronation. Reliable estimates directly link overpronation to 75 percent of all running injuries. This excessive movement strains supporting ligaments and tendons in the foot, leg, and knee. Supination or underpronation is the result of a high-arched rigid foot and is prone also to a variety of injuries. (See Figure 10.4).

Some doctors believe faulty anatomical structure, such as a too-short first metatarsal, can be blamed for some foot weaknesses. Other causes of weak foot are overweight, muscle strain, disease, congenital defects, inactivity or excessive use, and injury. Use Chart XII in the Appendix for a foot evaluation.

SHIN SPLINTS

Shin splints are a dull throbbing pain on the shin bone. No one really knows what causes them. Some theories are that shin splints are caused by changing running surfaces (hard to soft), running on hard surfaces, bringing the foot over too much in front of the other one when running (putting pressure on the fibula), wearing improper shoes, being overweight, or using the feet and legs in an unaccustomed manner such as overuse or improper use. Some pathological theories are that the muscle has pulled away from the bone, the membrane between the tibia and fibula is stretched, or that there are microscopic tears in the muscles.

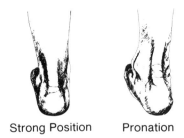

Strong Position   Pronation

FIGURE 10.4 Normal and abnormal foot alignment

Shin splints are more likely to occur in a person whose muscles are weak. The only cure is rest. Several different treatments might alleviate the pain, such as the application of cold or heat, massage, or a combination of these. Shin splints are a very individual condition; thus what works for one person may not help another. Stretching the calf muscles and strengthening the anterior tibial muscles may help prevent shin splints. Stretching the shin muscles before and after, jogging may also help prevent or alleviate the pain. Many people tape the tibia and fibula together but, this is not a good practice since it can retard circulation to the foot.

SELECTED FOOT EXERCISES

Toe Curling—Alternate flexing and extending of toes improves circulation (a big factor in preventing varicose veins) and strengthens the arches.

Walking Barefoot in the Sand—This is a good exercise for foot muscles.

Outward Roll—Stand with the feet slightly apart and roll the weight toward the outside borders of the feet. Repeat 10 times.

Walk on Tiptoes—Walk with the feet toeing in (pigeon toed) for 50 steps.

Marble Pickup—Pick up marbles or an imaginary object with your toes. Repeat 10 times.

Achilles Stretch—Stand with the toes and balls of the feet on a thick book. Lower the heels to the floor. Repeat 10 times. Hold 10–30 seconds.

Foot Circling—Sit, or lie supine, with the legs extended. Point the toes of the feet downward, turn the soles toward each other, bring the toes toward the shins (dorsiflex). Repeat 10 times.

Towel Grip—Sit on a stool or chair and place a towel on the floor. Keep the feet parallel (about 10 inches apart) and under the knees. Grip the towel with the toes and gather it into a mound while keeping heel on floor.

Isometric Inversion—Sit in a chair with one ankle resting on the other thigh. Supinate the foot while resisting with the hands. Hold for six seconds; repeat three times with each foot.

Shin Stretch—Sit in chair and extend both legs in front of body, keeping feet flat on floor, force the ankles into plantar flexion, stretching the anterior tibialis.

Ankle Flex—Sit in a chair with feet about six inches apart and flat on the floor. Roll ankles in, then out, as far as possible. Raise each heel alternately as high as possible while keeping toes on the floor. Raise each ball of foot alternately as high as possible while keeping heel on floor. Repeat pattern 10 times.

REFERENCES

1. *Runner's World* "Shoe Issue" (October 1986 pp. 31–34) and April 1987 p. 47.
2. *Runner's World,* April 1987, pp. 39–40.

Relarxation

11

PRETEST

1. Is stress always bad?
2. What are the effects of stress and neuromuscular hypertension?
3. What are well-known methods of relaxing? *massage, recreation, rhythmic, stretching*
4. What is diaphragmatic breathing?

Relaxation may be defined as the release of neuromuscular tension. It is a skill which can be learned and practiced and is as important an aspect of total fitness as is strength. Unfortunately, it is an aspect too often neglected. With the present-day emphasis on contracting muscles, we forget to learn how to "uncontract" them.

We are faced daily with tension-building situations in this fast-paced modern world. The game of the century is "Beat the Clock"—competition under pressure, and a race against time. We build up tension from worry, fears, anxiety, and physical and mental fatigue. We need ways to prevent or release these tensions; therefore, relaxation plays a vital part in contributing to one's health.

TENSION

Tension is necessary in order to be awake and alert. It is a general condition of activity in the body—a state of "readiness" for response on the part of the muscles, organs, glands, and nerves. What we are concerned about is *excess* tension: specifically, *residual neuromuscular hypertension.* Failure to release unnecessary tensions because of inadequate rest and sleep, and the inability to relax will result in a chronic state of fatigue and excess muscle tension. This muscle tension may cause backaches, headaches, or difficulty in getting to sleep. Heart attacks, ulcers, menstrual irregularities, nervous, and psychic disorders may be related to conditions of tension.

Tension may manifest itself in nervous mannerisms such as fidgeting and finger tapping; or in static positions such as clenched teeth, frowning, hunched shoulders, and a tight fist. Incoordination and inefficiency, as well as psychosomatic ailments such as headaches and digestive upsets, may be symptomatic of neuromuscular hypertension.

Dr. Roy Menninger, a noted psychiatrist, stated that 70 percent of the population are affected from time to time with "problems of living."[1] He contends that stress need not be bad for people. Many persons actually thrive on stress. The problem is learning to cope with stress. Dr. Menninger says that people must recognize stress and train themselves to withdraw psychologically from the circumstances.

Prevention of Neuromuscular Hypertension

Much tension can be avoided by proper planning of your daily life—balancing work and rest. "Moderation in all things" may still be a helpful adage. At the first sign of fatigue, when you feel yourself becoming irritable, take a "breather." Provision should be made for recreational activities and diversions which promote the release of inner stresses. Whether it be a rousing game of tennis, gardening, or music, one needs a "safety valve" to prevent built-up tension. Good body mechanics can help to prevent tension, since efficient movement requires the use of only those muscles essential to the task, preventing unnecessary energy expenditure and strain.

Methods of Releasing Tension

Alcohol, tranquilizers, pain pills, and other drugs are *not* the answer. Begin by trying to find out why you are tense, and strive to remove the cause. Some people can relax more easily than others; but releasing tension is a matter of self-discipline and can be learned.

Recreation, in the out-of-doors if possible, is strongly recommended as both a sedative and a cathartic. Massage and heat are soothing and comforting. Mild, rhythmic exercise routines can be beneficial. Stretching exercises to pull the tightness out of muscles are good if done slowly and held for a moment. Try rolling your head in a half circle (not backward). As a break from your studies, lie with your feet elevated and your neck supported by a rolled-up towel for 10 to 15 minutes.

It is not uncommon to find it difficult to reduce body tensions enough to fall asleep at night. Some suggestions for preventing this "wide-eyed" feeling are:

1. Go to bed at a regular time.
2. Avoid eating *heavy* foods before bedtime.
3. Start "letting down" at least 45 minutes before retiring.
4. Take a warm shower.
5. Eliminate distractions such as light and noise.
6. Drinking milk

CONSCIOUS TECHNIQUES OF RELAXATION

A conscious relaxation of at least 20 minutes a day is remarkably helpful. Use of such a technique before falling asleep will help insure falling asleep more quickly, and result in a sounder, more restful sleep. There are a number of well-known "methods" of relaxing, and while these systems differ somewhat, most of them offer suggestions similar to these:

1. Learn to recognize neuromuscular tension in a body part and the feeling of releasing it by deliberately tightening a muscle and then "letting it go." Relaxing is said to be zero activity—not something you do, but rather, something you cease to do.
2. Lie on your back in a comfortable position, and concentrate on your breathing without changing its rhythm. Gradually extend the exhalation, and as you do so, consciously release the muscular tension in your body.
3. Try to "let go," and continue "letting go" beyond the point of zero tension. Start at the toes (or some other body part) and work up to the legs, thighs, abdomen, lower back, upper back, arms, neck, shoulders, chest, face, mouth, jaw, and tongue. It is easier to relax the large muscle groups (arms, legs, trunk, and neck), but with practice, the small muscles (face, mouth, and tongue) can also be controlled.
4. Success may not be immediate, but it will come with practice. As skill is acquired, you may be able to release tension in the body as a whole rather than concentrating on individual body parts.
5. Use a "sort-of" self-hypnosis, imagining yourself on a feather bed or floating on a cloud; or visualizing yourself as a rag doll or a heavy bag of sand, with the sand slowly sifting through a hole in the sack.

With practice, and the acquisition of the kinesthetic perception for tension and the release of tension, conscious relaxation can be used in almost any situation where tension builds up in your daily life. Lying, sitting, or standing, you can learn to relax isolated body parts or the entire body when the situation demands and without others noticing your technique. Whether it be final examination jitters or stage fright before an audience, the ability to relax will make your adjustment to life more successful.

SELECTED RELAXATION EXERCISES

Arm Swings
Stand with the feet apart, arms at your side; inhale and raise the arms slowly forward to shoulder height. Exhale, and release all muscular tension in the arms, allowing them to drop to the sides and swing passively until all momentum is spent.

Repeat as above, except after the arms drop and swing down and backward and rebound forward, raise them again as you inhale. Repeat pendular relaxed swings in rhythm with your breathing.

Leg Swings

Stand on one leg, with the hip on the opposite side elevated so that the leg can swing freely, just brushing the floor with your foot. Execute leg swings the same as arm swings, using a minimum of muscular contraction, with tension only as the forward momentum is spent and the leg is raised to hip level. Keep the lower leg relaxed and the knee bent on the forward lift.

Trunk Swings

Stand with your feet apart and the knees slightly bent. Bend forward at the hips, and let the head, neck, arms, and trunk dangle toward the floor. With a minimum of muscular effort, set the trunk swinging from side to side by shifting the weight from one foot to the other, letting the heels come off the floor alternately. Then, with a slight springing movement of the lower back, gently bob up and down, keeping the entire body limp.

Shoulder Drop

Sit tailor fashion on the floor, or sit in a chair with arms relaxed. Tip your head forward, and let it hang relaxed. Inhale and hunch one shoulder, then let it drop as you exhale; repeat with the other shoulder; repeat with both shoulders at the same time.

Diaphragmatic Breathing

Lie on your back with your knees bent. Relax. Place your hands on your abdomen and breathe through your nose naturally. Feel your hands rise and fall. Concentrate on your breathing. After your breathing becomes slower, try pulling your diaphragm up at the end of the exhalation.

REFERENCE

1. Sorochan, W. *Promoting Your Health.* New York: John Wylie & Sons, Inc. 1981. p. 58.

Special Exercise Concerns for Women

12

[handwritten annotations: Structural causes - place of uterus. functional causes - tension, depression, anxiety; poor posture, fatigue, tension, constipation, lack of muscle tone, sluggish circulation]

PRETEST

1. What is dysmenorrhea?
2. What are the symptoms of PMS?
3. How do you prevent osteoporosis?
4. Why is it important for pregnant women to continue to be physically active?

Women have some unique health concerns which may raise questions about when and how to exercise. In most cases, exercise of the proper kind can prevent or alleviate problems as well as help maintain good physical fitness. This chapter will discuss the role of exercise in menstruation, pregnancy, and osteoporosis.

MENSTRUATION

Menstruation, which begins at puberty and ends at menopause, is a series of events occurring in a cycle. Normally a woman will menstruate four to six days at 20- to 30-day intervals, but it varies with the individual. Five days at a 28-day interval is average. The purpose of the menstrual cycle is to prepare the uterus for nurturing a new life and to eliminate that preparation if the ovum is not fertilized. The walls of the uterus become engorged with blood and nutritive elements to supply the fertilized ovum with a means of growth. This cannot return to the blood stream and so is lost by a direct flow from the uterus.

The entire cycle is a normal process and should not be painful. However, there are normal biochemical changes occurring in the body during menstruation, such as increased congestion in the pelvic area, heightened irritability, lowered threshold for pain, more susceptibility to environmental temperature changes, and decreased flexibility (especially in the lower back and pelvic regions). Common symptoms, preceding and during the menstrual flow, may be one or more of the following: protruding abdomen, enlarged breasts and soreness, weight gain, and pain (cramps, headache, leg ache, nausea and low back pain). Changes in one's daily routine, such as emotional upsets and new living arrangements, can result in minor fluctuations in the cycle.

PREMENSTRUAL SYNDROME

Premenstrual Syndrome (PMS) is a combination of physical and/or emotional symptoms that occur before menstruation and disappear or decrease during and after menstruation. The timing, when the symptoms begin, varies with individuals, but they usually appear at midpoint in the premenstrual cycle.

The exact cause of PMS is unknown. Many researchers believe that it is related to hormonal and biochemical changes that accompany the menstrual cycle, and psychological factors may also play a role. PMS does not occur during pregnancy, after menopause, or following surgical removal of the ovaries. There is a wide variety of symptoms for PMS. Some are tension, depression, irritability, headache, breast tenderness, fluid retention, backache, dizziness, abdominal cramps, weight gain, fatigue, mood swings, increased appetite, and food cravings.

Because no single treatment is uniformly effective, each woman must be treated individually. Symptomatic treatment is the best that can be offered. Fluid retention causing swelling and bloating may be helped by limiting the salt intake and perhaps using a diuretic. Aspirin or acetaminophen helps alleviate some symptoms as does dietary modification. Avoiding sugar, tobacco, and excessive consumption of alcohol the week prior to the menstrual period is suggested. The hormone progesterone has been used extensively but its value and safety are debated. The same is true with vitamin B_6 (pyridoxin). (See chapter 6.) Exercise may help since it is known to have an antidepressant effect. Caffeine worsens PMS in some and improves it in others.

If you seek treatment for PMS, you should be cautious and skeptical. Do not hesitate to get a second opinion as treatment for PMS has become a profitable business.

DYSMENORRHEA

Dysmenorrhea (painful menstruation) is not normal, but approximately one-half of the women who menstruate have menstrual discomfort with some regularity. Many have severe pain that incapacitates them for a day or two each month. It is one of the most common causes of lost work and school hours in the country. Loss of work time because of this so-called "feminine handicap" has been a problem for both employers and employees.

There are two general types—structural and functional. Structural dysmenorrhea arises from such things as malformations, endocrine imbalance, or malpositions and should be referred to your family doctor for diagnosis and treatment. Innumerable theories have been advanced as to the causes of functional dysmenorrhea: defective posture (especially swayback), fatigue, tension, constipation, lack of muscle strength, and sluggish circulation due to lack of exercise. Gynecologists estimate that 70 to 80 percent of the cases of painful menstruation are functional.

Recent research has determined that there are at least 10 prescription drugs that are effective in the majority of cases of dysmenorrhea. These are anti-prostaglandin drugs. Indications show that dysmenorrheic women often have high levels of hormone-like proteins called prostaglandins. According to current thinking, raised levels of prostaglandins produced by many tissues of the body (including uterus lining) cause contractions, lack of oxygen, and nervous sensitivity which create dysmenorrhea in some women. Prostaglandin inhibitors are marketed primarily as anti-inflammatory drugs for arthritis. Since these drugs are taken for so short a period, the side effects so far have been minimal. Aspirin also inhibits prostaglandins, but is much weaker than the prescription drugs. Any woman with severe menstrual cramps should discuss this treatment with her physician.

You may prevent or find relief from minor pain by:

1. Improving your daily health habits through an adequate diet and a balance of activity and rest.
2. Improving poor posture.
3. Exercising regularly and using special remedial exercises.
4. Wearing proper clothing (avoid tight belts and girdles).
5. Applying heat to the lower back and abdomen.
6. Learning to relax (see chapter 12).

A large majority of gynecologists place no restrictions on the usual daily routine, including vigorous activity (such as swimming) and intensive sports competition during all phases of the cycle. Normal hygiene practices should be carried on—bathing, shampooing hair, etc. It is extremely important that you observe care in your personal cleanliness while menstruating because you may perspire more and body odors are more offensive at this time—even your breath may carry a distinctive menstrual odor.

SELECTED EXERCISES FOR DYSMENORRHEA

Many exercises or physical activities that improve circulation and lower back flexibility may prevent dysmenorrhea or give relief. A few of the exercises, some named for the gynecologists by whom they were prescribed, are described here:

Billig Exercise—Stand with your left side to the wall, heels and toes together; left arm bent at a right angle, forearm and hand resting on the wall at shoulder level parallel to the floor. Place the right hand on the right hip; and "push" the hips slowly and steadily toward the wall, keeping the back erect, lower back flat, and the knees extended. Do this three times to the left and three times to the right. Repeat three times a day.

Mosher Exercise—Assume a hook-lying position, with the right hand resting on the abdomen. Raise the lower abdomen as high as possible (balloon), keeping the lower back flat on the floor. Lower the abdomen by pulling in and up and contracting your abdominals. Repeat 10 to 20 times. Do not hold your breath but continue to breathe normally.

Knee-Chest Position—Kneel with the thighs perpendicular to the floor, rest the cheek on the floor, and place your arms at your sides or place your hands under the cheek. Maintain this position for 10 to 15 minutes.

Mad Cat Exercise—On hands and knees with head raised permit the abdominals "to drop" and the back to sway. Then drop the head and flatten the abdomen by "pulling it in," and "hump" the back, holding for a count of five. Relax for five counts and repeat three or four times.

OTHER MENSTRUAL CONDITIONS

Toxic Shock Syndrome

Although rare, this syndrome is of concern to some tampon users. This disease is caused by a bacterium, Staphylococcus Aureus. The part tampons play in this is not yet known. Medical consultants suggest that if you use tampons do not use them continually; use menstrual pads at night and on days of light flow.

Secondary Amenorrhea

Cessation of the menstrual flow has appeared in females who do intense and frequent aerobic work bouts. Many female distance runners, those who run 10 to 15 miles per day, experience this condition, as do some dancers and cyclists. The reason for this is not known, but one theory postulates that there is a correlation between secondary amenorrhea and lowered percentage of body fat. Usually when the intensive work bouts cease, the menses returns. If this does not happen, see your physician immediately.

OSTEOPOROSIS

Osteoporosis means increased porosity of bone. It is a condition in which bone structures degenerate due to loss of calcium. Normally bone density and strength peak at about age 20. After age 30–35, women lose three-fourths to one percent of bone mass each year until menopause, then lose two to three percent for five years. Men, starting at age 50, lose bone at a rate of four tenths percent a year.

Osteoporosis affects 20 million Americans, mostly women over 45 years of age and is the leading cause of death among older women in the United States, due to bone fractures and subsequent complications such as pneumonia. It is eight times as common in women as in men. It usually occurs after menopause or a hysterectomy, so the reduced amount of estrogen seems to be a factor. There is no cure, so prevention is the key.

The general recommendation is exercise regularly, do not smoke, and do eat foods rich in calcium and vitamin D. Vitamin D and fluoride help the body absorb calcium. Before going on a calcium or vitamin D supplement, you should consult your physician since too much calcium can cause kidney problems and high blood pressure. Excessive amounts of vitamin D can lead to vitamin D toxicity. Calcium intake is easily met by consuming dairy products and dark green leafy vegetables. Equally important is exercise. Bearing weight on long bones and stressing bones by the pull of muscles during exercise slows bone loss significantly and may even increase bone mass. If you have weak bones because of poor diet and insufficient exercise, as you lose calcium you could become an invalid and lose five to seven inches in height and become "hump" back. Excessive intake of protein, fiber, alcohol, and caffeine cause loss of calcium along with phosphorous as found in many soft drinks.

EXERCISES DURING PREGNANCY

Normally, you should continue to be phsycially active during pregnancy. Exercise during this period and after giving birth is as essential to good health as under ordinary circumstances. With regular exercise, you will not only feel better but also be better prepared for the delivery of your baby. Many daily activities such as sitting, standing, walking, stair climbing, kneeling, and squatting are good forms of exercise. Since these activities compose a much greater percentage of your movements during the day than a regular exercise routine, they should be performed with efficient body mechanics. You should consult your doctor before undertaking or continuing an exercise program during pregnancy.

An exercise regime can benefit you in many ways: strengthening muscles, improving flexibility, increasing overall muscle strength, weight control and learning to relax. Maintaining your own exercise program may be easier for you than learning a new activity. Be sure to include warming-up and cooling-down periods, breathe normally, and do only exercises where the hips are kept lower than the heart. The latter exercises cause a build-up of pressure in your thoracic cavity which puts additional work on the heart and lungs. Avoid exercises that will stress your abdominals and those that include sudden twisting. Women with normal pregnancies can safely exercise at 60 percent of their maximal heart rate.

Selected Exercises for the Pregnant Woman

Leg Extensor—Assume a hook-lying position. Slowly slide the right leg down, keeping the sole of the foot and the base of the spine on the floor as long as possible. Extend the leg fully, and then slowly slide the leg to the initial position. Repeat three to five times with each leg. Inhaling as the foot slides up and exhaling as it slides down.

Knee Raise—Assume a hook-lying position. Bring the right thigh toward the chest, keeping the knee bent. Return to the initial position, and repeat with the other leg. Repeat three to five times with each leg, inhaling as the thigh comes up and exhaling as it goes down.

Frog Kick—Lie supine. Place soles of feet together by rotating legs outward. Draw the legs upward until the outsides of the knees are touching, or almost touching, the floor. Extend legs downward, keeping the soles of the feet together as long as you can. Repeat slowly three to five times, inhaling as legs are drawn upward and exhaling as they are extended.

Hip Raiser—Assume a hook-lying position, with arms at sides. Slowly raise the lower part of the spine off the floor as the body weight is shifted toward your knees and heels as if trying to get up. Gradually return to the initial position, leading with the lower part of your spine. Repeat three to five times, inhaling as the spine is raised and exhaling as it is lowered.

Back Relaxer—Assume a supine position with arms at sides. Sit up; grasp your right knee, keeping the left leg extended. Keep the left leg on the floor as you rock back and forth five or six times, holding the right knee. Return to the initial position, and repeat with the left knee. Keep your back curved and your breathing effortless.

Leg Relaxer—Lie supine. Place your lower legs on a chair or stool of average height. Heels should be fully supported and the chair placed so that you have no feeling of holding up your legs. Relax. Take deep breaths through your nose and exhale through your mouth.

Ankle Flex—Lie supine with legs extended, arms at sides. Flex your ankles by pointing with the heels. Repeat 10 to 12 times, inhaling as you flex and exhaling on the return to initial position.

Arm Twist—Stand erect, facing a wall at about an arm's length. Place the palms of your hands on the wall directly in front of your shoulders. Lean forward slightly, resting your weight on both hands. Without moving, your hands, rotate the elbows until they point outward, and then return to initial position. Repeat slowly five or six times. Place your hands so that the fingertips point toward one another. Rotate the elbows downward and then return to initial position. Repeat slowly five or six times, exhaling as elbows go down and inhaling as they go up.

Glossary

Acute   Having a short and relatively severe course.

Anemia   Having too few healthy red blood cells or too little hemoglobin in the red blood cells.

Angina pectoris   Condition marked by recurrent pain in the chest and left arm caused by a sudden increase of the blood supply to the heart muscle.

Anorexia nervosa   A psychological disturbance causing an abnormal desire to lose weight and an excessive concern about appearance leading to a pathological fear of becoming fat.

Arteriosclerosis   Thickening and loss of elasticity of the artery walls.

Atherosclerosis   Same as arteriosclerosis.

Atrophied   Decreased in size; wasted away.

Basal metabolism rate (BMR)   Magnitude of heat loss while one is lying down.

Blood pressure (BP)   Pressure of blood within the arteries when the heart is relaxing. Expressed in two figures; for example, 120/80 of which systolic is the higher and diastolic is the lower.

Body composition   Percentage of fat in the body, ratio of fat to lean tissue.

Bulemia   A psychological condition causing a syndrome of overeating (binge) followed by vomiting (purge) in a repeated cycle.

Cardiac output (Q)   Volume of blood ejected into the main artery by each ventricle, usually expressed as liters per minute.

Charlatan   A faker or fraud or quack; one who pretends to a knowledge they do not have.

Cholesterol   Special type of fat associated with saturated fats; it causes atherosclerosis by lining the walls of arteries.

Chronic   Lasting a long time or recurring often.

Coccyx   Small triangular bone at the lower end of the vertebral column; tail bone.

Crunches   Partial situps; curl-ups.

Diabetes   Metabolic disorder in which the body cannot use carbohydrates efficiently.

Diastolic pressure   Phase of the blood pressure when the heart is relaxed and filling for the next contraction (just before a ventricular contraction).

Diaphragmatic breathing   Inhaling deeply so chest rises.

Double-blind study   Research study technique in which neither the subjects, nor the experimenter knows who is getting the experimental treatment (or drug) until after the data are collected.

Dynamic   Physical force in motion; movement of the joints is involved.

Fallacies   False or erroneous ideas.

Fibula   Long thin outer bone between the knee and ankle.

Gluteals   Buttocks muscles.

Gluttony   Excessive eating or drinking.

Hamstrings   Posterior upper leg muscles.

Heart rate (HR)   Number of ventricular beats per minute.

Hormone   Chemical substance produced in the body to regulate other body functions

Huckster   One who hawks or peddles a product or service with showmanship.

Human chorionic gonadotropin   Hormone extracted from the urine of a pregnant woman.

Hypertension   Abnormally high blood pressure, or a disease of which this is the primary sign.

Hypocalcemia   Abnormally low level of calcium in the blood.

Lactation   A mother secreting milk for nursing her baby.

Maximal oxygen uptake (Max $\dot{V}O_2$)   Highest oxygen uptake that one can attain during physical work; sometimes referred to as maximum aerobic power.

Megadose   Very large dose, much greater than normal dose.

Metabolic rate   Magnitude of heat production as assessed by the measurement of oxygen uptake.

Neuromuscular hypertension   Excess tension in skeletal muscles.

Obesity   Excessive body fat resulting in a significant health impairment.

Oxygen uptake ($\dot{V}O_2$)   Volume of oxygen extracted from the inspired air usually expressed as liters per minute.

Pectorals   Arm muscles which attach on the chest.

Polyunsaturated fat   Essential fatty acids; most of the vegetable oils (unless hydrogenated).

Premenstrual syndrome (PMS)   Combination of physical and/or emotional symptoms that occur before menstruation and disappear or decrease during and after menstruation.

Pronation   Bearing the weight on the inner border of the foot.

Prone   Lying in a face down position.

Pulse rate   Frequency of pressure waves (waves per minute) propagated along the peripheral arteries (such as the carotid and the radial).

Quack   One who pretends to a skill or knowledge they do not have.

Sacrum   bones of the lower spine (above the coccyx).

Shin splin   ⅊ll throbbing pain of the shin (front of lower leg).

Stroke v   ⅊V)   Amount of blood ejected into the main arteries by each
    ver   r beat.

Subcuta   Below (underneath) the skin.

Supinat   ⅉearing weight on the outer border of the foot.

Supine   g in a face up position.

Systol   **ure**   Phase of the blood pressure when the heart contracts (ven-
    ⅉject blood into the pulmonary and systemic arteries).

Tensi   ⅉate of "readiness" of the body.

Ther   ⅉsis   Body's mechanism for resisting weight gain.

Tibi   er leg bone between the knee and ankle; shin bone.

To   Poisonous.

Tri   ⅉes   Fatty substance (manufactured from carbohydrates) in the
    d stream that is a major constituent of very low density lipoprotein
    ⅉDL).

V   Pertaining to blood vessels.

ⅉ   ⅉs   Two lower chambers of the heart which receive blood from the
ⅉper chambers and pump it into the arteries.

Index